The

SIBO
SOLUTION

+ **40**
RECIPES

**YOUR COMPREHENSIVE
GUIDE TO ELIMINATING
SMALL INTESTINAL
BACTERIAL OVERGROWTH**

Sylvie McCracken

Sylvie McCracken of HollywoodHomestead.com

About the Author

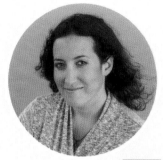

SYLVIE IS A NUTRITION AND HEALTH EDUCATOR, SHARING HER LATEST ARTICLES AND RECIPES ON HER POPULAR BLOG, HOLLYWOODHOMESTEAD.COM

You can find out more about their lifestyle at the blog hollywoodhomestead.com and follow her on Facebook, Twitter, Pinterest, and Instagram.

Sign up for the newletter at: hollywoodhomestead.com/sign-up

She is the author of two other books (available on her website): Paleo Made Easy: Getting your Family Started with the Optimal Healthy Lifestyle and The Gelatin Secret: The Surprising Superfood that Transforms your Health and Beauty

Holding a Bachelor of Science in Finance, business is one of her first true loves which is why she recently launched a second website (SylvieMcCracken.com) to help others start and grow their own online businesses.

She's also a wife and mother of three children ages 4 through 16. Last year she wrapped up a decade-long career as a celebrity personal assistant in Hollywood and moved to Abu Dhabi where her husband will be teaching for a couple of years.

Sylvie and her husband Eric each lost over 60 lbs in the first year of adopting a paleo diet. You can read about their paleo success stories on HollywoodHomestead.com

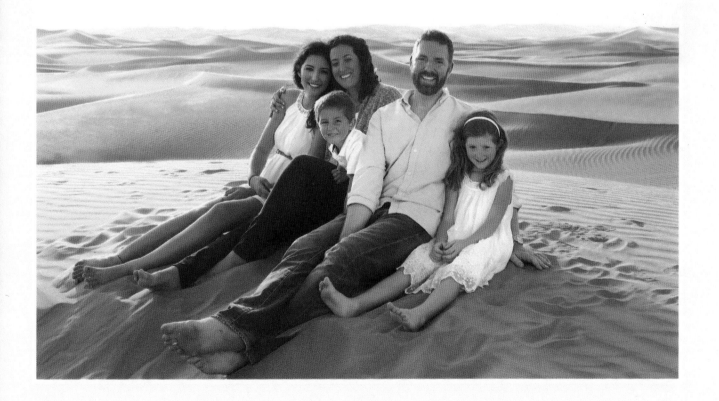

Contents

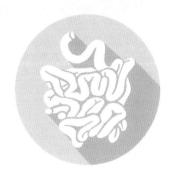

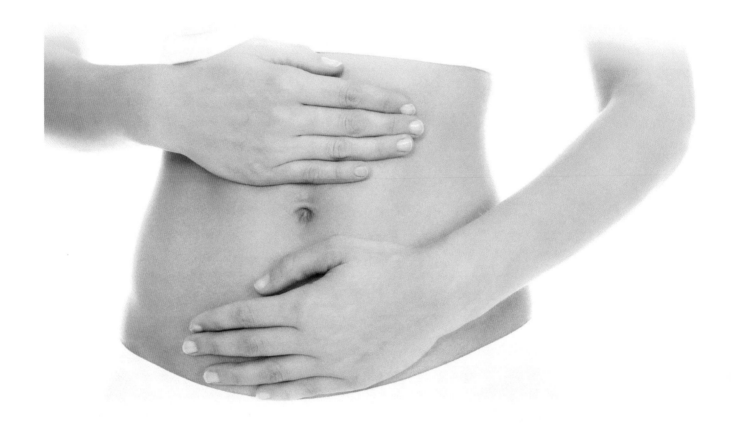

Introduction

IF YOU'RE READING THIS BOOK, MY GUESS IS THAT YOU, LIKE ME, HAVE BEEN DIAGNOSED WITH SIBO (SMALL INTESTINAL BACTERIAL OVERGROWTH). OR PERHAPS YOU'RE SIMPLY CURIOUS ABOUT WHETHER YOU HAVE SIBO BASED ON YOUR DIGESTIVE SYMPTOMS. EITHER WAY, YOU'VE COME TO THE RIGHT PLACE.

In this book you will learn all about what SIBO is, what causes it, how to *accurately* diagnose it, treatment methods, and how to make sure it never comes back! I also have lots of great SIBO friendly recipes for you to promote healing and prevent recurrence.

WHY DID I DECIDE TO WRITE ABOUT SIBO?

As with most of my work, it started as a struggle. When I was first diagnosed with SIBO, I was actually relieved because I'd been jumping from one doctor to another bringing with me articles about SIBO and asking them to test me for it since it seemed like a very likely possibility based on my symptoms. The fist doc just rolled his eyes. The second doc told me to go ahead and assume I have SIBO and, without bothering to test, wrote me a prescription for an antibiotic which I reluctantly accepted. It didn't work. Turns out (as you and I now both know) SIBO can't be fixed by simply taking a pill. Luckily my third doc agreed to test me and sure enough, by then I had a severe case of methane dominant SIBO, the hardest to treat. How long I had it or what the cause was is still a bit of a mystery.

Of all the diagnoses I've had over the years, SIBO has been by far the most frustrating one and the most complex to treat. Except for a few specialists, most doctors are not very knowledgeable on this subject and many are quick to dismiss it as something of nominal importance. Some think it doesn't even exist and that you should just treat the symptoms and quit your whining. Even in the hands of a SIBO specialist, such as the ones at the SIBO center in Portland, Oregon, there's only so much that can be done in a 30 or 60 minute consultation and the bulk of it is in your hands between appointments.

Does this sound familiar to you? I understand your frustration. I understand what it's like to want to feel well. I also understand how demoralizing it is when you finally start eating healthy foods and get sicker instead of getting better.

As a side note, it is pretty ironic that certain healthy foods (like fermented foods) are bad for SIBO. Yet, if we'd eaten these foods from the get-go, they could have *prevented* SIBO (such as by building a strong immune system and gut flora). The fact that you've got to eliminate lots of healthy foods from your diet to heal SIBO is downright maddening! And if someone that doesn't understand SIBO hears you say you can't eat apples or garlic because they're a FODMAP (see page <u>62</u> for more info on FODMAPs) they'll likely try to have you committed ;)

In writing this book, my goal isn't just to offer you sympathy and understanding. I also want to give you hope. I was able to eradicate my severe case of SIBO, and you can too. I know it. I also know it will take a hefty dose of hard work and determination.

I hope that The SIBO Solution can serve as your guidebook to navigate you through diagnosing the condition, understanding treatment options, a prevention strategy, and your diet. Your health is your hands and you deserve it.

¹ What is SIBO?

NOT THAT LONG AGO, THE WORD "BACTERIA" BROUGHT UP ALL SORTS OF NEGATIVE CONNOTATIONS AND WE'D DO ANYTHING TO KEEP IT OUT OF OUR BODIES. THEN WE STARTED TO REALIZE HOW IMPORTANT SOME TYPES OF BACTERIA ARE FOR OUR BODIES. HENCE, THE BOOM OF PROBIOTIC SUPPLEMENTS AND TRENDY YOGURTS. BUT IT ISN'T ADEQUATE TO LABEL BACTERIA SIMPLY AS "GOOD" OR "BAD." A TYPE OF BACTERIA MIGHT BE "GOOD" IN ONE PART OF YOUR BODY, BUT "BAD" IN ANOTHER. LIKEWISE, TOO MUCH "GOOD" BACTERIA CAN BE A VERY BAD THING. THIS IS WHAT HAPPENS WITH SIBO—SMALL INTESTINAL BACTERIAL OVERGROWTH SYNDROME. LET'S START WITH THE BASICS ...

WHAT IS SIBO?

SIBO is a bacterial infection of the small intestine. Now, bacteria is normal in the digestive tract so that's not the problem. But, with SIBO, it isn't the presence of bacteria which is the problem. The problem is that there is *too much* bacteria and/or *the wrong type of bacteria and it's in the wrong place.* By the "wrong type of bacteria," it doesn't necessarily mean some weird strain of bacteria is wreaking havoc on your gut. Most often, SIBO occurs because bacteria which should be in your *large intestine* gets into your *small intestine or simply isn't moving down to your large intestine as it should.*[1] SIBO is not contagious so you don't have to worry about it spreading to anyone else.

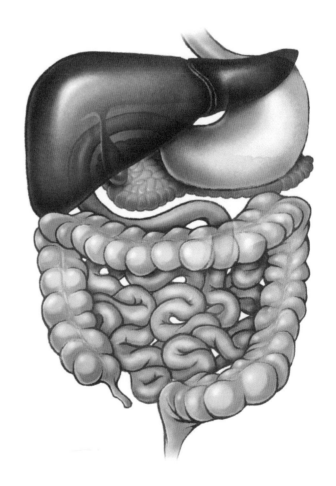

UNDERSTANDING THE DIGESTIVE SYSTEM

Before we can talk about what SIBO is and why you should be worried about it, we need to go over how the digestive system works. When you eat, food passes through your body in a series of tubes. At each stage, there are various acids which break down food so your body can absorb nutrients.

- **Mouth:** Chewing and saliva start breaking down starches.

- **Esophagus:** Swallowing brings food to the stomach.

- **Stomach:** Muscle movements mix food with stomach acid.

- **Small Intestine:** Food mixes with stomach acids, bile from the liver, and pancreatic juices. Food is broken down and absorbed through the walls of the small intestine.

- **Large Intestine:** The large intestine takes waste from the small intestine. It absorbs any remaining nutrients. It also absorbs liquid so the waste turns into stool. The stool is then pushed out of the body during a bowel movement.

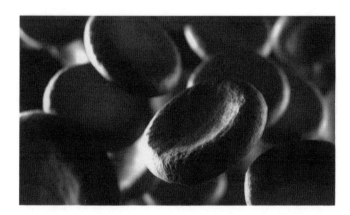

The small intestine is really quite fascinating. It is about 3.5 times your body height—or about 20 feet long![2] Aside from the first few inches of the small intestine which are smooth, the small intestine is made up of many folds called *mucosal folds*. It is also lined with finger-like projections called *villi*. The folds and villi increase the surface area of the small intestine so it can better absorb nutrients, sort of like a towel with increased surface area helps you absorb water. The folds also help your small intestine mix food with acids so they can be broken down.

The small intestine is arguably the most important part of the digestive process. It is in the small intestines that food is broken down into absorbable parts. The small intestines are responsible for getting these nutrients into our bloodstream so we can use them.[3,4]

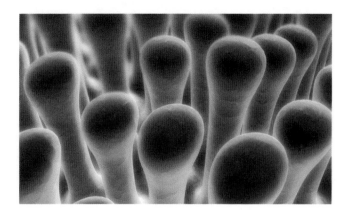

The Role of Gut Bacteria

Before you get scared off by the idea of bacteria in your digestive tract and take steps to eliminate all of it, you need to be aware that we need bacteria. There are about 100 *trillion* bacteria in our intestines alone! This is about 10 times the number of cells our bodies have.

Bacteria in the gut has numerous functions, including:

- Breaking down carbohydrates so they can be absorbed;

- Helping the gut's immune system develop;

- Protecting against disease-causing bacteria;

- Stimulating the growth of the intestinal lining;

- Converting vitamin K_1 into vitamin K_2, which is an important nutrient for bone health.[5]

Bacteria is so important for our health that it is now often referred to as "the forgotten organ."[6]

The vast majority of bacteria in our guts is located in the large intestine. To put this in perspective, there are about 10–100 billion bacteria organisms present per teaspoon of fluid in the large intestine, compared to just around 100 thousand organisms in the small intestine.[7]

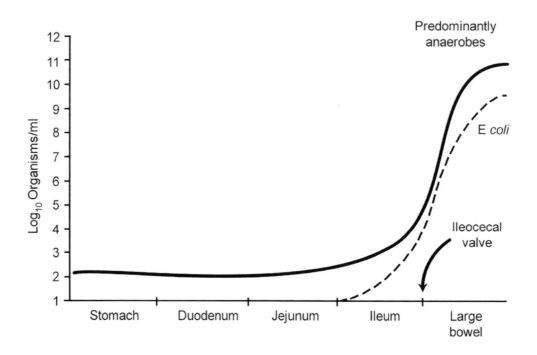

Concentration of bacterial flora in different parts of the gastrointestinal tract

The location and concentration of bacteria throughout the intestines is really important for health. With SIBO, the problem is NOT that you have bacteria in your small intestine. The problem isn't even one type of bacteria. The problem is that you have:

i. Too much bacteria and/or

ii. The wrong types of bacteria

It is thought that SIBO is most commonly caused when bacteria which should be in the large intestine (and would be harmless there) gets into the small intestine. However, it is also possible for SIBO to be caused by an overgrowth of the normal bacteria which should be in the small intestine. This may occur when there is a problem with the Migrating Motor Complex which acts as a housekeeper to sweep bacteria out of the small intestine, which we talk more about in chapter 13 about prokinetics.[1]

This is why SIBO is so hard to treat. If it were just a problem of one type of bacteria, or too much bacteria, then we could take antibiotics and kill off the "bad" bacteria. But SIBO involves multiple types of bacteria, including normal "healthy" bacteria which *should* be present—just that it is present in the wrong part of the body and in too high of concentrations. While antibiotics are a great life-saving innovation, they are commonly overprescribed and very ineffective for treating SIBO.

Taking antibiotics may get rid of the overgrowth temporarily, but they can upset your gut flora balance and the "bad" bacteria is just likely to proliferate again—which is why SIBO recurrence is so high. Because antibiotics also kill off the healthy bacteria which should be in your gut, taking antibiotics can ironically be a cause of SIBO! If you do use antibiotics to treat SIBO, they MUST be combined with and followed by a strict diet for prevention as well as prokinetics. Otherwise, recurrence is almost inevitable. We will get more into this more in the chapters about treating SIBO and diet protocols.

² Symptoms of SIBO

AS YOU'D EXPECT, SIBO CAUSES MANY GASTROINTESTINAL SYMPTOMS. HOWEVER, BECAUSE THE GUT IS LINKED TO VIRTUALLY EVERY OTHER PART OF THE BODY, SIBO CAN CAUSE A WIDE RANGE OF SYMPTOMS FROM DEPRESSION TO SKIN RASHES.

GI SYMPTOMS OF SIBO

When you have too much bacteria in your gut, the bacteria will start feeding off of undigested particles of food. The bacteria causes the starches to ferment. The fermentation process produces hydrogen gas as a by-product. If you have an overgrowth of bacteria, then the bacteria are going to have a field day eating away at your food—before your body can even start digesting them. You end up with a gut full of hydrogen gas.

With the methane-producing type of SIBO (which we will get into in chapter 08), there is also an overgrowth of archaea, which are single-cell organisms without a nucleus. The archaea feed off of hydrogen, but they produce methane as a byproduct. In either case, you end up with a lot of gas in your gut.

What happens when your gut is full of gas? Well, the obvious symptoms are that you are going to have flatulence and/or belching. The gas can also cause severe bloating. Even if you are thin, the bloating can be so bad that you look like you are 5 or more months pregnant.

Another problem which sometimes occurs with SIBO is severe abdominal pain. This is partly due to the fact that the intestines are sensitive to pressure, so even a small amount of gas can cause pain. The pain can also be caused by *visceral hypersensitivity.* Dr. Christina Lasich describes visceral sensitivity very well by comparing it to a sunburn. When your skin becomes burned, even the slightest touch makes it hurt. This is hypersensitivity. Well, the very same thing can happen when your gut is chronically damaged, making the pain more intense.[8]

Two common symptoms of SIBO are either diarrhea or constipation and sometimes alternation between the two. Hydrogen-producing SIBO is associated with diarrhea. Methane, which slows down motility (the transit of substances through the bowel), is associated with constipation. However, it is possible and common even to have both hydrogen and methane present, so having alternating bouts of both diarrhea and constipation are not uncommon SIBO symptoms.[9]

> ### GI SYMPTOMS OVERVIEW:
> - **Flatulence and/or belching**
> - **Bloating**
> - **Abdominal pain**
> - **Cramps**
> - **Diarrhea and/or constipation**

OTHER SYMPTOMS OF SIBO

If it were just digestive problems that we were talking about, then SIBO wouldn't be such a big deal. But our gut is responsible for much more than just eating. It's not for nothing that experts refer to it as our second brain. Problems in the gut can cause other problems including malnutrition, neurological and psychological problems, and skin problems.

Malnutrition from SIBO

Digestion starts the moment you put something in your mouth. Chewing starts to break down starches and saliva further breaks them down. Powerful acids in your stomach break down proteins. Bile from the liver and pancreatic juices flow into the small intestine where they mix with stomach acids to break down carbohydrates, proteins, and fats. It is here in the 20 feet of small intestine that the bulk of digestion occurs. It is also in the small intestine that nutrients are absorbed.

SMALL INTESTINE

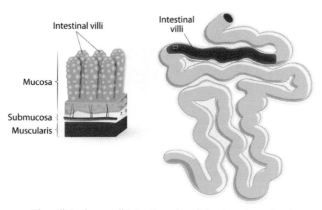

The villi in the small intestine absorb broken down food so we can get the nutrients we need.

For example, bile usually helps break down fats. When you have SIBO though, the bacteria deconjugate (disrupt) bile salts, leading to insufficient amounts of fat absorption. This is NOT a good thing! Your body relies on dietary fat to transport fat-soluble vitamins. This is why SIBO can cause deficiencies in vitamins A, D, and E. Vitamin K is also a fat-soluble vitamin. However, because it is produced from fermentation, vitamin K deficiency is rare in SIBO.[11]

THERE ARE TWO WAYS THAT SIBO CAUSES MALNUTRITION:

- **Bacteria compete for nutrients**

- **Bacteria produce byproducts which irritate and inflame the small intestine, hindering nutrient absorption**[10]

WHAT'S THE BIG DEAL WITH THESE VITAMIN DEFICIENCIES ANYWAY?

- **Vitamin A Deficiency = poor immune system, vision problems like night blindness**

- **Vitamin D Deficiency = poor bone health, hormonal problems, increased cancer risk**

- **Vitamin E Deficiency = muscle weakness, vision problems, poor immunity**[12]

The unabsorbed fatty acids can also cause other nutritional problems. The acids can bind with minerals like calcium and magnesium (important for bone health) and form "soaps" which your body can't break down. This drastically increases the risk of bone diseases.[13]

B_{12} deficiency is also a major problem with SIBO because the bacteria consume the B_{12} before the body can absorb it. It might seem like popping a few B_{12} supplements would solve this problem but, because people with gut disorders can also have trouble absorbing B_{12}, those oral supplements might not help. You'd need to take B_{12} injections or B_{12} as a nasal spray to fix the deficiency while working on your SIBO attack plan.[14]

B_{12} has many important roles, including making DNA and keeping the body's blood and nerve cells healthy. Without enough B_{12}, you can experience symptoms like:

- Fatigue
- Depression
- Confusion
- Poor memory
- Nerve problems like numbness or tingling
- Megaloblastic anemia[15]

And this is just the tip of the iceberg! Because the bacteria can inflame and damage the sensitive villi lining the small intestine, the body can have problems absorbing all sorts of nutrients. You can eat an incredibly healthy diet full of superfoods but it won't do you any good if your body can't absorb the nutrients!

Psychological Symptoms of SIBO

Recently, experts have come to recognize a strong connection between the brain and the intestines. They call this the gut-brain axis. The gut-brain axis is so powerful that our gut bacteria is now often referred to as the "second brain."[16]

The gut-brain axis isn't exactly a new discovery. For over 100 years, scientists have known that the brain can influence the gut. One example is the army surgeon William Beaumont who, in the 1830s, found that changes in mood affected gastric secretions in the gut. Even people without a medical background can recognize the gut-brain axis. Think about it: when you are stressed, you often get indigestion. When you are depressed, you often feel the urge to eat.

What is new information about the gut-brain axis is that researchers finally realized that it is a two-way street. Actually, more like a cylindrical street. The brain affects the gut, and the gut can affect the brain. For example, stress is thought to be a major cause of SIBO. But, a damaged gut can also affect your brain and make you feel stressed. That is why stress can be both a cause and a symptom of SIBO.[17]

The gut-brain axis is fairly complex, especially when you take into account that there billions of neurons in our brains, *trillions* of bacteria in our guts, and upwards of 1,000 distinct species of bacteria in the gut. Obviously, there is a lot to analyze!

The vast majority (90%) of the brain's output goes through the *pontomedullary* area of the brain stem, which then goes to the vagus nerve. The vagus nerve goes through the heart, esophagus, and lungs and into the gut.[17]

Studies now show that changes to gut microbiota can affect the brain. (*Microbiota, also known as gut flora, is a term which includes all microbes living in the gut, including bacteria, archaea, fungi, and viruses). The microbiota influence the brain even when the immune system isn't activated, which means it is the microbiota which are directly "talking" to the brain! Note though that it isn't just the microbiota itself which is doing the talking. Bacteria in the gut can cause inflammation, which is an immune response, and the immune system also communicates with the brain.[16, 18]

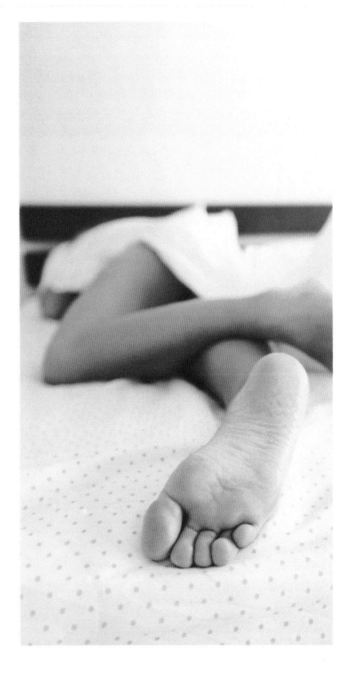

Most of the studies to date have been on animals, but the results are pretty amazing. For example, when rats were fed an antibiotic-laced drinking water, it caused anxiety-like behavior. When the antibiotic treatment stopped, their behavior went back to normal two weeks later.[16] The human studies which have been done mostly involve administering probiotics, and have found that probiotics can influence mood.[18]

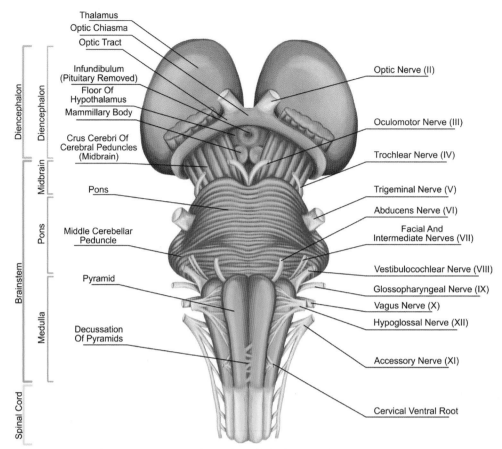

The vagus nerve goes down through the lungs and heart into the gut

Because of the gut-brain axis, these are some of the SIBO symptoms you might experience:

- Stress
- Brain fog
- Poor memory
- Anxiety
- Depression

Remember, the gut-brain axis is a two-way street. **Stress, neurological, and psychological problems aren't just *symptoms* of SIBO, but can also be *causes* of SIBO!**

To learn more about the brain connection with SIBO, I highly recommend reading Dr. Kharrazian's brain book called *Why Isn't My Brain Working*. In the book, he teaches you nutritional strategies for improving brain function, like how gargling several times a day for long-ish periods of time can stimulate your vagus nerve which improves blood flow to the gut. You can find the book on our resource page www.hollywoodhomestead.com/sibo-solution-resources/

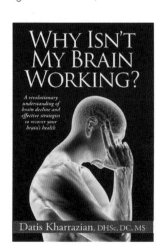

Skin Conditions as Symptoms of SIBO

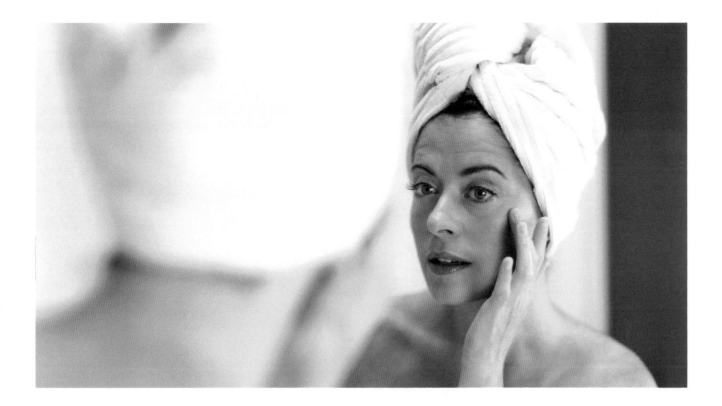

Do you have acne, rashes, or eczema? Or maybe you just have uneven, flaky skin? These can all be symptoms of SIBO. On a basic level, SIBO can cause skin problems because it interferes with nutrient absorption, and poor nutrition often reveals itself first through your skin. As talked about earlier, SIBO particularly interferes with the absorption of fat-soluble vitamins, including Vitamin E which is known for its role in skin health.

However, the main reason that skin conditions are a symptom of SIBO probably goes back to the gut-brain axis. Well, we need to add one more axis: *The gut-skin axis.* You have already experienced your brain-skin axis, such as when your skin flushes when you become em-barrassed or you get a breakout right before a stressful exam. Since the gut influences the brain, it follows suit that the gut can influence your skin.

Interestingly, the gut may be able to influence the skin directly. Your skin is teeming with bacteria: there are about 1 million bacteria living on each square inch of skin you have.[19] Research indicates that signals from your gut bacteria can interact directly with the bacteria on your skin.[20] The bacteria in SIBO can also cause inflammation, which also is a trigger for acne.

Like with the gut-brain axis, much more research is needed before we can fully understand the gut-skin axis. However, we do know these facts:

- A study found that SIBO is 10 times more prevalent in those with acne rosacea vs. healthy controls (people without acne)

- Correction of SIBO leads to marked clinical improvement in patients with rosacea

- A Russian investigation reported that 54% of acne patients have marked alterations to the intestinal microflora

- A Chinese study involving patients with seborrheic dermatitis also noted disruptions of the normal gastrointestinal microflora[21]

³ Causes of SIBO

OBVIOUSLY, SIBO IS CAUSED BY HAVING TOO MUCH BACTERIA IN YOUR SMALL INTESTINE. HOWEVER, WHEN TALKING ABOUT THE CAUSE OF SIBO, WE CAN'T PUT THE BLAME ON THE BACTERIA ITSELF. REMEMBER, YOU ARE *SUPPOSED* TO HAVE BACTERIA IN YOUR GUT AND SIBO IS MOST OFTEN CAUSED BY AN OVERGROWTH OF BACTERIA WHICH *SHOULD* BE THERE. INSTEAD OF BLAMING BACTERIA AS THE CAUSE OF SIBO, THE REAL CAUSES ARE THE THINGS WHICH MADE THE BACTERIA PROLIFERATE IN THE FIRST PLACE.

In this chapter, we will talk about the main underlying causes of SIBO. It is important to understand these causes so you can take steps to eliminate them. Otherwise, your SIBO will probably just come back after treatment.

STRESS

The majority of SIBO cases are likely caused by stress.[1] Stress is also what makes SIBO so likely to come back after you treat it. As we talked about in the chapter about symptoms, the gut is linked to the brain in what is called the gut-brain axis. Without rehashing all of the info found in that chapter, researchers have now discovered that it isn't just our brains which communicate to the gut, but *bacteria in our gut "talk" to the brain.*

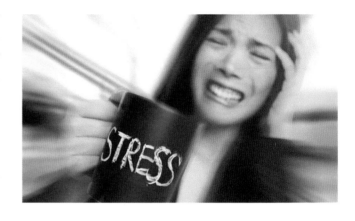

If you take a group of healthy people, they each will have different bacterial compositions in their guts. Yet, each person's gut bacteria stays pretty much the same—even when compositions are measured months or more apart. But, when you take a person and put him in a stressful situation, the bacterial composition drastically changes. This creates an imbalance in bacteria which can affect health.[16]

Stress can also indirectly cause SIBO by creating conditions which lead to SIBO.

- Stress → Inflammation → **Low Stomach Acid** → **SIBO**

- Stress → Weakened Immunity → **Overgrowth of "Bad" Bacteria** → **SIBO**

- Stress → Weakened Immunity → **Infection** → **Antibiotic Use** → **SIBO**

- Stress → Motility Problems → **Bacteria Proliferation** → **SIBO**

Remember, the gut-brain axis is a two-way street! This is why stress can be both a *cause and symptom of SIBO.* To cure SIBO for good, it isn't enough to take antibiotics and make changes to your diet. You've also got to manage stress.

ANTIBIOTICS

As someone who took entire arsenals of antibiotics during the first 2 decades of my life (including large doses of penicillin injected into my rear more times than I can count!), I can attest to how quick doctors are to prescribe antibiotics. In Argentina where I grew up, you can even get antibiotics without a prescription. I would just call my doctor who lived in another province and tell him my symptoms. He'd tell me what antibiotics to pick up, increasing my dosage each time. Now, I'm not anti-doctor nor anti-medicine by any means and I think antibiotics can be a great, even life saving, tool in some instances but using them as a first recourse for things that could have been treated with some chicken soup and a little rest doesn't come without consequences.

It isn't just in Argentina were antibiotic over-prescription is a problem. One survey found that American medical doctors prescribe antibiotics in about 101 million visits yearly![22] Other studies have found that these antibiotics are often unnecessary—such as when they are given when the underlying problem is actually a virus.[23] It also doesn't help that antibiotics are regularly given to livestock animals, which is another reason to buy antibiotic-free meat.[24] Actually, if you want to improve your gut and overall health, buy pasture raised meat which has a better Omega-3 to Omega-6 ratio. For bonus points, visit the farm to confirm the quality! Overuse of antibiotics leads to antibiotic-resistant superbugs, which is a major threat to health. To learn more about the importance of meat quality for health, I recommend reading my first book, *Paleo Made Easy*, which can be found on the resource page www.hollywood-homestead.com/sibo-solution-resources/. But let's just look at what antibiotics can do to our gut health.

When you take antibiotics, they don't just kill off the "bad" bacteria which are causing your infection. They kill off the "good" bacteria which need to be in your gut. This upsets the balance of your gut flora. Without enough good bacteria to keep the bad bacteria in check, the bad bacteria can proliferate and lead to SIBO.

Once you consider the link between antibiotic use and SIBO, it is easy to understand why SIBO has such a high recurrence rate. Doctors traditionally prescribe antibiotics for SIBO, which temporarily may solve the problem. However, the *antibiotics do not address the underlying cause of SIBO*. Because the healthy bacteria are also affected when you take antibiotics for SIBO, the bad bacteria just proliferate again and SIBO comes back. This is why it is so important to follow diet and lifestyle protocols to prevent SIBO recurrence.

LOW GASTRIC ACID

Acid reflux is incredibly common: 50% of adults will experience some type of gastroesophageal reflux disease in a 12 month period and 20–30% will have weekly symptoms.[25] Based on all those heartburn medicine ads you see on TV, you would think that acid reflux is caused by having *too much gastric acid* and that antacids are the solution to all your problems. Really, heartburn is caused by *too little acid*.[26]

The symptoms of acid reflux do not occur from having too much acid, but rather occur when acid gets into the esophagus. This can happen when there is too much pressure (such as from inflammation and excess stomach gas) and the pressure causes stomach acids to be pushed up into the esophagus. Antacids do wonders for suppressing the *symptoms* of acid reflux but, because you *need acid*, they don't address the underlying problem and actually make the problem worse in the long run.[27]

Our bodies need gastric acid to digest food and break it down. Without enough stomach acid, you end up with undigested carbohydrates in your digestive tract. Bacteria in your small intestines love most carbohydrates and they start to feed off of them. Not only do the bacteria proliferate, leading to SIBO, but the bacteria produce hydrogen gas as a byproduct of digesting carbs. You end up with a belly full of gas, which in turn creates intra-abdominal pressure and pushes your stomach acid up into your esophagus—causing acid reflux.

According to researchers Suarez and Levitt, just **1 ounce of carbohydrates that escapes absorption in a day could produce more than ten quarts of hydrogen gas in small intestine.** This gives you an idea of how much pressure undigested carbs can produce![28]

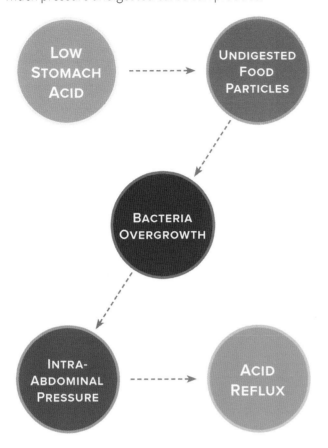

Gastric acid not only helps digest food, but also suppresses ingested bacteria naturally. So, low gastric acid is a double-edged sword. Bacteria proliferate because there is so many undigested carbs to feed off of, and they continue to proliferate because there isn't enough gastric acid to suppress growth.[29]

WHY WOULD YOU HAVE LOW STOMACH ACID?

The obvious answer to this question is that you have been prescribed proton pump inhibitors or are taking antacids for acid reflux. But what caused you to have the acid reflux symptoms in the first place?

Though the drug industry would rather you didn't know about it, research shows that ulcers are caused by a bacteria called *h. pylori* which is present in as many as ⅔ of the population.[30]

There are many other reasons why your stomach acid production might be low. Some of these include old age, stress, adrenal fatigue, chlorinated water, and alcohol consumption.[31] A big contributing factor though, is diet. The junk foods and carbs which make up the Standard American Diet are very inflammatory. As Dr. Myhill explains:

"The stomach is lined with cells that are proton pumps—that is to say they pump hydrogen ions from the blood stream into the lumen of the stomach. Stomach acid is simply concentrated hydrogen ions. There is a natural tendency for these hydrogen ions to diffuse back from where they came but this is prevented by very tight junctions between stomach wall cells. However, if the gut becomes inflamed for whatever reason, there is leaky gut and hydrogen ions leak back out."[32]

YOU MAY HAVE LOW STOMACH ACID WHICH CAUSED SIBO IF:

- **You have h. pylori infection**
- **You have leaky gut syndrome (mainly caused by food sensitivities like gluten)**
- **You take proton pump inhibitors or antacids regularly**

In this way, SIBO is linked to leaky gut syndrome, which is the cause of all autoimmune disorders.

Poor Immunity

Our immune systems are a heck of a lot smarter than antibiotics at controlling "bad" bacteria. A healthy immune system will control bacteria in the small intestines by secreting mucus containing immunoglobulins. When your immune system becomes compromised, SIBO can occur. SIBO has been linked to many immunodeficiency syndromes.[11]

Instead of asking how impaired immunity causes SIBO, we should be looking at the root cause: *why is your immune system not functioning in the first place?* Of course, there are many possible reasons for this, such as stress and poor diet. Do you see a recurring theme here? Stress and poor diet are at the root of most causes of SIBO!

Dysmotility

Another major cause of SIBO is dysmotility, which is a condition in which the muscles of the digestive system become impaired and are no longer able to empty contents efficiently. The contents become trapped in the small intestine. Motility is incredibly important for protecting against SIBO: the movements in the bowl prevent organisms from attaching to the wall of the small intestines. When you've got food waste sitting in your small intestines instead of exiting through the large intestine, bacteria can start to proliferate as it feeds on the waste.[11]

The movements of our digestive system are actually on a rhythmic schedule which is known as the *migrating motor complex* (MMC). It is thought that MMC has a "housekeeping" role. One of the biggest mistakes I made when first attempting to treat SIBO was not immediately taking a prokinetic after treatment. A prokinetic is different than a laxative, which stimulates *peristalsis,* or the movement of food through the gut. Prokinetics are what stimulate the MMC to empty food residue and bacteria left in the small intestine.[33] We will talk about prokinetics and improving motility in chapter 13.

Dysmotility can be a genetic problem. In genetic cases, it is common for family members to also have other muscle contraction problems, such as incontinence from not being able to control the bladder. Dysmotility can also be caused by problems like:

- Parkinson's Disease
- Diabetes
- Scleroderma
- Thyroid disorders
- Lupus
- Amyloidosis
- Muscular dystrophy
- **Inflammation of the intestines**[34, 29]

This last point is very important. Note the recurring theme. Stress and bad diet can cause gut inflammation. This can then led to low stomach acid, which in turn leads to bacterial overgrowth. This in turn leads to more stress, which creates a vicious cycle. Again, this is why it is so important to treat SIBO with a comprehensive strategy which includes diet and stress management.

Heavy Metals as a Cause of SIBO

Another possible cause of SIBO is heavy metals toxicity. Every day, we come into contact with a barrage of toxic heavy metals. For example:

- Aluminum found in toothpaste, baking soda, and aluminum cans
- Cadmium in drinking water, plastics, and paint
- Lead in car exhaust, eating utensils, and canned foods
- Mercury in air conditioner filters, overconsumption of certain fish, and floor waxes
- Arsenic in wine, household detergents, and preservatives

Even if you take steps to eliminate heavy metals from your life (such as by making your own toothpaste and cleaning products), it is still impossible to completely avoid toxic heavy metals. These heavy metals have been shown to have adverse effects on your body, including on your digestive tract.[35, 36]

Even "healthy" heavy metals can be harmful to your gut health. For example, iron and some other nutrients are considered heavy metals but your body needs them to function. But, if your gut is damaged (such as from inflammation and leaky gut), then you won't be able to absorb these nutrients into your body. "Bad" bacteria use some heavy metals to form *biofilms*. Biofilms are basically mesh-like structures where bacteria live. To form biofilms, bacteria use iron, calcium, and magnesium (amongst others). The biofilm acts as a shield which protect the bacteria and makes it very difficult for probiotics or antibiotics to kill the bacteria. This is obviously a Catch-22 because you need those metal nutrients to stay healthy, but they also can help the bad bacteria thrive.[37]

ON A PERSONAL NOTE ...

The truth is that I don't know 100% what the cause of my SIBO was. For me, there were probably numerous underlying causes of my SIBO ... chronic antibiotic use in my formative years, a damaged gut from the junk food diet I used to eat, heavy metal exposure (I tested high for mercury and lead to be specific), h. pylori, chronic stress ...

SIBO can be a vicious cycle. It is caused by stress. Trying to figure out SIBO makes you more stressed. The SIBO comes back and you get more stressed.

Understanding that cycle is the easy part. Breaking it is the tricky part.

All of the causes above are issues that I have personally struggled with. It is hard to pin down, but you've got to do your best to attack SIBO with a multidimensional approach. Just taking antibiotics probably won't cure you if you don't make major changes to your lifestyle and diet. The good news is that, once you master these changes, it isn't just your gut health which will be better—you entire health and happiness will improve.

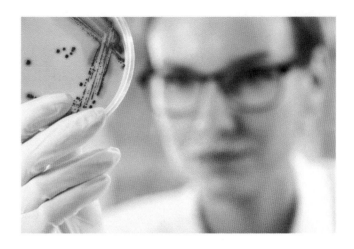

CARBOHYDRATE MALABSORPTION

Carbohydrate malabsorption, also called carbohydrate intolerance, is a condition in which your body is unable to digest or properly absorb certain carbohydrates. There are numerous carbohydrate intolerances but some of the most common are fructose, lactose, sucrose, and sugar alcohols (such as sorbitol and xylitol). When the body is unable to digest these carbs properly, bacteria are able to use it as food and proliferate. As with many things related to SIBO, carbohydrate malabsorption can be a vicious cycle. Not only is it a potential cause of SIBO, but SIBO can cause malabsorption problems—thus giving bacteria more carbs to feed off of and worsening the SIBO.[38, 29]

"A wonderful, easy to read book by a fellow (former) SIBO sufferer. I was honored to be a part of her journey".

— **DR ALLISON SIEBECKER**, OREGON

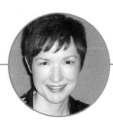

⁴Prevalence of SIBO

IT WAS ONLY RECENTLY THAT MEDICAL RESEARCHERS DISCOVERED JUST HOW IMPORTANT THE GUT IS TO OUR OVERALL HEALTH. SO, IT ISN'T SURPRISING THAT THE GUT WAS (AND STILL IS) OFTEN OVERLOOKED. TO PUT THIS IN PERSPECTIVE, CONSIDER THAT CROHN'S DISEASE WASN'T EVEN DESCRIBED UNTIL THE 1930S. IRRITABLE BOWEL SYNDROME (IBS) WASN'T MENTIONED UNTIL THE 1950S. IT TOOK EVEN LONGER FOR THESE DISEASES TO GET MUCH RECOGNITION IN POPULAR MEDICINE.[39, 40, 41]

By comparison, SIBO is even newer. It wasn't until 2004 that the link between SIBO and constipation was discovered. In recent years, interest and research in SIBO from the medical community has greatly increased—but don't be surprised if your doctor seems amazingly unaware of the disease and treatment protocols.[42]

I mention all this to point out that *we really don't know how prevalent SIBO is.* If your doctor isn't aware of it, then he/she probably isn't going to order a breath test, let alone the *right* breath test as discussed on page 30. Even if you are given a breath test, your doctor might only order a hydrogen test instead of a hydrogen *and* methane test (you've got to do both tests; we will discuss why in chapter 06 about diagnosing SIBO). There are still no established protocols on how to read the results of SIBO breath tests, so one doctor might give a negative diagnosis whereas another might diagnose positively.

There also have been very few studies on the prevalence of SIBO in seemingly-healthy subjects (there have been ample studies about the occurrence of SIBO in patients with IBS and other GI disorders). Further, the prevalence rates also depend on what diagnostic method is used. Even with these limitations in research, it is pretty clear that SIBO is a very common health problem, even in "healthy" people.

One analysis of SIBO research from 1966 to 2006 found these prevalence rates in "healthy" groups:

- 0% (glucose breath test)
- 5.9% (glucose breath test)
- 13% (lactulose breath test)
- 14.5% (glucose breath test)

- 20% (lactulose breath test)[29]

I find it interesting that the one study which found a 0% rate of SIBO was in Japan. The other studies were in westernized countries like the US, UK and Australia. The Japanese are known for their really low obesity rates, their long lives, and a gut-healthy diet which traditionally doesn't include any wheat (gluten). It makes you think...

In a different analysis of the literature, SIBO prevalence was found to be:

- 0–12.5% by the glucose test
- 20–22% by lactulose test
- 0–35% by xylose test [43]

Keep in mind these statistics are for *healthy* subjects. When you look at the prevalence rates of SIBO for people with IBS, Crohn's or other gut problems/symptoms, then prevalence rates skyrocket. For example, one research paper found that 36% to 84% of patients with IBS also have SIBO. Consider that IBS affects 10–15% of the North American population and you can see how big of a problem SIBO may turn out to be.[44]

Note also that the research clearly shows that advanced age is a risk factor for SIBO. Up to 35% of "healthy" elderly adults have been found to have SIBO.

THE BOTTOM LINE?

If you've got digestive issues, don't hesitate in testing for SIBO. Insist on a hydrogen and methane **3 hour lactulose** breath test. If your doctor is reluctant to order one, then consider switching doctors! ∎

⁵ Associated Diseases

I REALLY WANT TO STRESS THAT THE GUT IS LINKED TO VIRTUALLY EVERY PART AND SYSTEM OF YOUR BODY. WE DON'T JUST HAVE THE GUT-BRAIN AXIS, WE'VE GOT THE GUT-SKIN AXIS, GUT-LIVER AXIS, GUT-KIDNEY AXIS, GUT-BONE AXIS ... SINCE YOUR GUT IS WHAT IS RESPONSIBLE FOR TAKING IN NUTRIENTS AND GETTING THEM INTO YOUR BLOODSTREAM, YOUR GUT IS ALSO GOING TO BE LINKED TO ANY NUTRIENT DEFICIENCY DISORDER.

If you've got SIBO, you've got more than just a grumbling tummy and bloat to worry about!

Because of the gut's connection to every part of the body, we could potentially link SIBO to virtually every disease out there. At her website, Dr. Siebecker has a list of 50+ of these diseases and conditions, such as (to name just a few):[45]

- Acne Rosacea and Acne Vulgaris
- Anemia
- Autism
- Chronic fatigue syndrome
- Gallstones
- GERD
- Hypothyroidism
- Pancreatitis
- Rheumatoid arthritis

However, there are some diseases which are particularly associated with SIBO. They are *Irritable Bowel Syndrome, Crohn's Disease, Celiac Disease and Histamine Intolerance.*

IRRITABLE BOWEL SYNDROME (IBS)

IBS is an incredibly common disease which affects about 10–15% of the US population, and 9–23% of the population worldwide. The disease can affect anyone, but is most common in women. Having IBS is definitely no picnic. The symptoms are nearly identical to those of SIBO: abdominal pain, bloating, diarrhea and/or constipation, nausea, fatigue ...[46]

There has been quite a bit of research on the occurrence of SIBO in IBS patients. The results can't be ignored: upwards to 84% of IBS patients test positive for SIBO with a hydrogen breath test![45]

There seems to be a very strong link between SIBO and IBS, but medical professionals aren't in agreement on what exactly this link is. One possibility is that many people diagnosed with IBS really have SIBO. This is backed up by the fact that treatment for SIBO often gets rid of IBS symptoms. Another possibility is that SIBO is a root cause of IBS (no one knows for sure what causes IBS).[10]

However, some are skeptical of the link between SIBO and IBS. People with IBS have a shorter transit time from the stomach to the small intestine, which could cause a false positive on breath tests.[47]

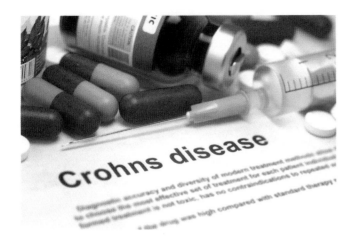

CROHN'S DISEASE

Crohn's Disease is an autoimmune condition in which the gastrointestinal tract is chronically inflamed. Crohn's most often affects the end of the small intestine, but can occur anywhere throughout the GI tract. This disease is definitely not something you want to have. It causes symptoms like persistent diarrhea, abdominal pain, rectal bleeding, and constipation.[39]

The cause of Crohn's Disease isn't fully understood, but scientists think it has to do with an immune response. Our immune systems generally do a great job of protecting our bodies against invaders like viruses, bacteria and fungi. With Crohn's Disease though, the immune system might mistakenly think that bacteria which normally should be in our GI tract is actually harmful. The immune system attacks these harmless bacteria, causing an inflammatory response.[39]

Because SIBO is a disease in which you've got too much or the wrong kind of bacteria in your gut, and Crohn's may be caused by gut bacteria, it isn't surprising that the two conditions are linked. Studies have found that 23–34% of Crohn's patients also tested positive for SIBO.

The theory is that Crohn's Disease predisposes people to SIBO because Crohn's causes motility problems. Disrupted motility means you have undigested food particles and waste sitting in your gut for longer, allowing bacteria to feast and grow.[48]

CELIAC DISEASE

Celiac Disease is finally getting a lot of attention and the world is waking up to the fact that gluten is not a friend of your gut. But the truth is that we may not know as much about Celiac Disease as we think. It is thought that Celiac is an autoimmune disorder. When people with Celiac eat gluten, the immune system attacks the gluten as though it were a foreign invader. This leads to inflammation which damages the lining of the small intestine.

There is another theory about the cause of Celiac Disease though.

Before gluten was even discovered, it was thought that SIBO was the cause of Celiac Disease. The first person to propose this theory was Dr. Sidney Haas in his 1951 book *The Management of Celiac Disease*. Dr. Haas treated over 600 cases of Celiac Disease using the Specific Carbohydrate Diet (which we will discuss in the diet chapter). In each case, he noted that prognosis was excellent.[49, 50]

One study found that ⅔ of Celiac patients who still had GI problems even after eliminating gluten tested positive for SIBO.[50]

It is worth noting that the only way to diagnose Celiac Disease is with an endoscopic biopsy, not a blood test. During the endoscopy, a scope is inserted through the mouth and down into the esophagus, stomach and small intestine. A sample of tissue is taken from the lining of the small intestine to look for damage to the villi.[51]

Even if you don't have Celiac Disease, gluten can still be a problem. Many people have a food sensitivity to gluten (called non-celiac food sensitivity). Depending on which study you go by, around 7–29% of people are sensitive to gluten, though some experts believe everyone is sensitive to gluten to some degree. The condition causes many of the same symptoms as Celiac Disease, including the inflammation which can lead to a damaged gut. Gluten sensitivity can be diagnosed with a blood test which looks for the presence of certain antibodies.[52, 53]

Gluten is definitely not good for your gut and can cause holes to form, so eliminating gluten might help elevate GI symptoms. But if you've been diagnosed with Celiac and still have problems even after eliminating gluten, you should get tested for SIBO and start following The SIBO Diet, not just a gluten-free diet.

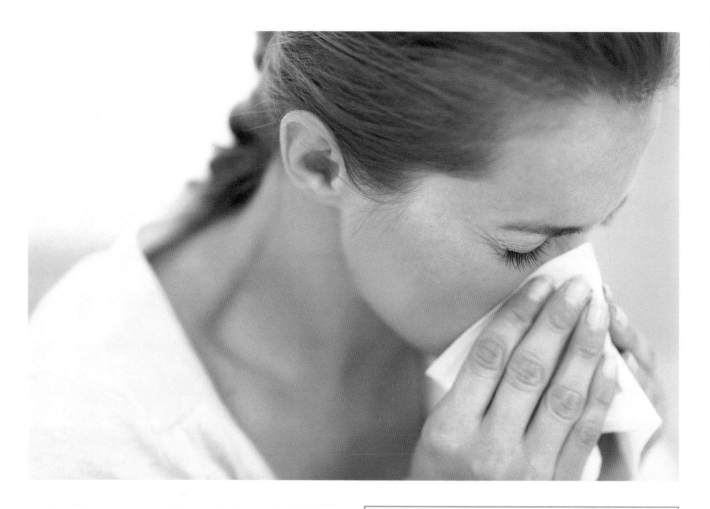

Histamine Intolerance

Histamine intolerance (HIT) is another condition which is also closely linked to SIBO. We tend to think of histamine as the chemical which our bodies release during an allergic attack, but histamine also has many roles in our body such as regulating stomach acid and immunity. Histamine is also found naturally in many foods. When you have HIT, your body has more histamine than it is able to break down and you experience allergy-like symptoms. Many practitioners, such as Chris Kresser, believe that HIT is caused by SIBO. Certain types of bacteria produce histamine from undigested food, causing excess histamine and symptoms. Finding out that histamine intolerance and SIBO are closely linked was the final clue that made me seek testing because my HIT was so bad at the time.[109]

"I absolutely love Sylvie's books and SIBO Solution is no different. Chock full of personal anecdotes and practical tips, this book is a must read for anyone suffering with major digestive distress or SIBO. Instead of this being a daunting or discouraging diagnosis, Sylvie gives us hope that there is a SIBO solution!"

She has a gift for distilling science and rigorous research into a language all of us can understand.

— **GENEVIEVE PAZDAN,** MamaNatural.com

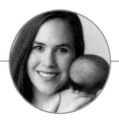

How to diagnose SIBO

WHEN YOU HAVE SIBO, YOU CAN EXPERIENCE A WIDE RANGE OF SYMPTOMS FROM GAS AND FLATULENCE TO FATIGUE AND DEPRESSION. IT IS IMPOSSIBLE TO DIAGNOSE SIBO BASED ON SYMPTOMS ALONE BECAUSE THE DISEASE SHARES SO MANY SYMPTOMS OF OTHER GUT DISEASES. THERE IS ALSO A STRONG LINK BETWEEN SIBO AND OTHER GUT DISEASES SUCH AS IRRITABLE BOWEL SYNDROME AND CELIAC DISEASE.

So, even if you have already been diagnosed with a gut disease which accounts for your symptoms, it is still good practice to test for SIBO. There are numerous different ways of diagnosing SIBO, but some tests are much more reliable than others. Here we will go over the different ways to diagnose SIBO and which ones are best.

SMALL BOWEL ASPIRATE TEST FOR SIBO

This test used to be considered the "Gold Standard" for diagnosing SIBO. It involves putting a tube down the nose, through the stomach, and into the small intestine to take a sample of fluid. Bacteria from the fluid is then grown (cultured) to determine what type and how much bacteria are present.

This test is no longer considered a good method for diagnosing SIBO. For starters, it is invasive and definitely not a pleasant experience for the patient! It also requires a highly-skilled professional to perform, and is costly. These problems might be acceptable, except that culturing bacteria isn't even a very accurate method of diagnosing SIBO. According to research published in the journal *Science,* this method only reveals about 20% of the microbiota in the small intestine, so SIBO could easily be missed.[54, 55]

STOOL TESTS FOR SIBO

Stool testing *cannot* diagnose SIBO because it mostly reflects the large intestine, and not the small intestine. This doesn't mean that it can't be a valuable diagnostic tool though. A stool test can suggest whether there is a bacterial overgrowth in the large intestine. It can also show fat malabsorption which may occur due to SIBO. Further, stool testing can be used to diagnose or eliminate other potential gut problems, such the presence of specific parasites. Some of the markers which may be measured in a stool test are:

- Digestion and Absorption Markers (pancreatic elastase, pancreatic enzymes, putrefactive SCFAs.)

- Gut Immunology Markers (inflammation markers)

- Metabolic Markers (pH, bile acids, levels of short chain fatty acids …)

- Microbiology Markers (pathogenic bacteria, beneficial flora …)

- Parasitology (presence of parasites or their eggs)[56, 57]

Urine Organic Acids Tests for SIBO

Bacteria and fungi in your gut produce organic acids as byproducts. These organic acids are then excreted in your urine. The presence of certain types of organic acids in your urine can be an indication that you have an overgrowth of bacteria or yeast.

Urine tests can only indirectly tell you if you have a bacterial overgrowth. They cannot tell you where the overgrowth is occurring, and thus can NOT be used to diagnose SIBO. However, some experts like Chris Kresser prefer the test because it also contains other markers which are useful for diagnosis.[56, 58]

Breath Tests—the Best Method for Diagnosing SIBO

Because of the limitations with the other SIBO diagnostic tests, breath tests are now considered the best way to diagnose SIBO.

The bacteria in our guts feed off of certain carbohydrates. They produce gases as a byproduct, including hydrogen and methane. Some of the gases are then absorbed through the lining of the colon and get into our blood. From there, the gases make it to our lungs and are exhaled in our breath. The amount of hydrogen and methane in our breath can indicate whether there is an overgrowth of bacteria in the small intestine.

Breath tests also aren't perfect for diagnosing SIBO, especially because there is no consensus on how to interpret test results. However, since it is thought that the only source of hydrogen in the body is from bacterial fermentation of carbohydrates, the hydrogen breath test is likely the most accurate method of diagnosing SIBO. It also has the benefit of being cheap, easy, and non-invasive.[54]

Note that not all breath tests for SIBO are the same. In the next chapter, we will get into the details about what you need to know about breath tests for SIBO.

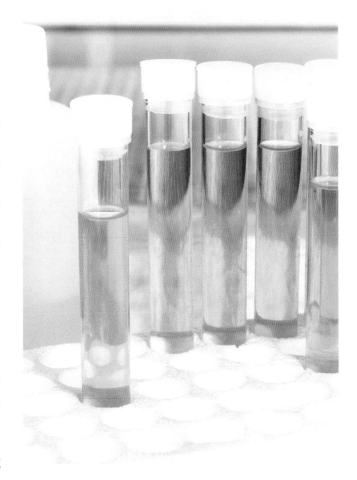

Diagnosing SIBO Doesn't Diagnose the Cause!

These diagnosis tests are simply used to tell whether you have an overgrowth of bacteria in your small intestine or not. Of course, this is important—but *the tests do not tell you what caused the SIBO in the first place.*

Bacterial overgrowth is an indication of an underlying problem. If you don't treat this root problem, then the SIBO is just likely to come back—regardless of how many rounds of antibiotics you take to kill the bacteria in your gut. Unfortunately, there are many possible reasons for SIBO. To really cure SIBO, you've got to take an multifaceted approach and make major lifestyle and diet changes so you don't create the conditions which allow your gut bacteria to become unbalanced.

Before and After SIBO Breath Test Results

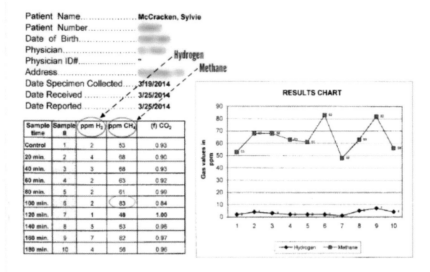

COMMONWEALTH LABORATORIES, INC.

Phone (800) 292-9019
FAX (781) 659-0705

39 Norman Street
Salem, MA 01970
customerservice@commlabsinc.com

Louis J. Traficante, Ph.D., DABFT
Laboratory Director

BACTERIAL OVERGROWTH REPORT SHEET 10 TUBE KIT

Patient Name.............................. McCracken, Sylvie
Patient Number..........................
Date of Birth..............................
Physician...................................
Physician ID#............................. "
Address......................................
Date Specimen Collected....... 3/19/2014
Date Received 3/25/2014
Date Reported 3/25/2014

Sample time	Sample #	ppm H₂	ppm CH₄	(f) CO₂
Control	1	2	53	0.93
20 min.	2	4	68	0.90
40 min.	3	3	68	0.93
60 min.	4	2	63	0.92
80 min.	5	2	61	0.99
100 min.	6	2	83	0.84
120 min.	7	1	48	1.00
140 min.	8	5	63	0.96
160 min.	9	7	82	0.97
180 min.	10	4	56	0.96

SUMMARY OF 2 HOUR RESULTS:

Peak Hydrogen Production:	3 ppm	Normal <20 ppm
Peak Methane Production:	35 ppm	Normal <20 ppm
Peak Combined H2 and CH4 Production:	38 ppm	Normal <20 ppm

BASED ON THIS STUDY BACTERIAL OVERGROWTH IS SUSPECTED.*

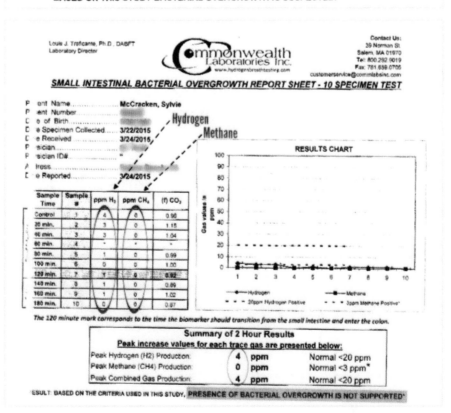

Louis J. Traficante, Ph.D., DABFT
Laboratory Director

Commonwealth Laboratories Inc.
www.hydrogenbreathtesting.com

Contact Us:
39 Norman St.
Salem, MA 01970
Tel: 800.292.9019
Fax: 781.659.0705
customerservice@commlabsinc.com

SMALL INTESTINAL BACTERIAL OVERGROWTH REPORT SHEET - 10 SPECIMEN TEST

Patient Name.............................. McCracken, Sylvie
Patient Number..........................
Date of Birth..............................
Date Specimen Collected....... 3/22/2015
Date Received 3/24/2015
Physician...................................
Physician ID#............................. "
Address......................................
Date Reported 3/24/2015

Sample Time	Sample #	ppm H₂	ppm CH₄	(f) CO₂
Control	1	4	0	0.96
20 min.	2	2	0	1.15
40 min.	3	3	0	1.04
60 min.	4	*	*	*
80 min.	5	1	0	0.99
100 min.	6	0	0	1.00
120 min.	7	1	0	0.92
140 min.	8	1	0	0.89
160 min.	9	1	0	1.02
180 min.	10	0	0	0.97

The 120 minute mark corresponds to the time the biomarker should transition from the small intestine and enter the colon.

Summary of 2 Hour Results
Peak increase values for each trace gas are presented below:

Peak Hydrogen (H2) Production:	4	ppm	Normal <20 ppm
Peak Methane (CH4) Production:	0	ppm	Normal <3 ppm*
Peak Combined Gas Production:	4	ppm	Normal <20 ppm

RESULT BASED ON THE CRITERIA USED IN THIS STUDY, **PRESENCE OF BACTERIAL OVERGROWTH IS NOT SUPPORTED***

⁷ Breath Tests for SIBO

IN THE LAST CHAPTER, WE TALKED ABOUT THE MANY WAYS TO DIAGNOSE SIBO. THOUGH THEY AREN'T PERFECT, BREATH TESTS ARE GENERALLY THE MOST RELIABLE AND AFFORDABLE METHOD OF DIAGNOSING SIBO. IT CAN BE A BIT CONFUSING BECAUSE THERE ARE NUMEROUS TYPES OF BREATH TESTS. HERE WE WILL TALK ABOUT WHAT BREATH TESTS ARE USED FOR, HOW TO TAKE A BREATH TEST, WHICH TYPE OF BREATH TEST YOU NEED TO TAKE TO DIAGNOSE SIBO AND HOW RESULTS ARE INTERPRETED.

WHAT ARE BREATH TESTS USED FOR?

The bacteria in our guts feed off of carbohydrates. They produce gases as a byproduct. Some of the gases are then absorbed through the lining of the colon and get into our blood. From there, the gases make it to our lungs and are exhaled in our breath. Thus, by measuring the levels and types of gas in our breath, we can get an idea of what and how much bacteria are in our guts.

Breath tests aren't just used to diagnose SIBO. They can also be used to diagnose H. pylori, lactose intolerance, and fructose intolerance among others. However, it is important to note that the breath tests are slightly different for each of these conditions. For example, the bacteria H. pylori produces carbon dioxide, so this is the gas that labs will be looking for in the breath test samples.[59]

To diagnose SIBO with breath tests, labs need to look for elevated levels of hydrogen and/or methane. Note that there is a difference between Hydrogen SIBO and Methane SIBO, which we will address in the next chapter.

HOW SIBO BREATH TESTS ARE PERFORMED

SIBO tests must be ordered by a doctor. You can take SIBO breath tests at home or you can perform them at the lab. You will be required to fast for at least 12 hours before the test is taken. That means no food, but prescription meds and water are okay. You may also need to stop taking certain supplements and antibiotics for two weeks prior to the test. You will also have to follow a special diet for 24 hours before the test. The diet basically removes any fermentable foods so you don't have gas in your GI tract prior to the test and get a false positive.

To take the test, you first breathe into a little tube (see picture) to measure your base hydrogen and methane levels. Then you immediately drink a special lactulose or glucose solution. You breathe into the tubes again every 20 minutes. To do it, you just breathe into them through a cocktail straw for a few seconds (as directed). You will see the condensation form. Then put the lid on and restart your timer. The test measures how the levels of hydrogen and methane change. A positive SIBO breath test is defined as one where there are peaks of hydrogen and/or methane after taking the sugar solution.[11]

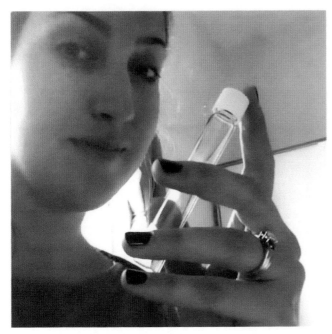

These are the tubes I had to breath in every 20 minutes for the SIBO breath test

LACTULOSE VS. GLUCOSE SIBO BREATH TESTS

Both lactulose and glucose are types of sugars. Not sugar as in the white stuff you buy in supermarkets, but sugar as in the substance that our bodies break carbohydrates down into. Bacteria digest the sugars and produce gas as a byproduct, which can be measured in a breath test. The difference between the two tests is that Glucose is only absorbed in the first three feet of the small intestine (remember, the small intestine is about 20 feet long!). **The glucose test cannot diagnose SIBO in the last 17 feet of the small intestine. SIBO is thought to be more common in the end parts of the small intestine, so the lactulose test is generally going to be more accurate for diagnosing SIBO.**[60]

There are also other breath tests available, such as one using the sugar xylose, but these aren't as reliable and may give a false negative.

YOU MUST TEST FOR BOTH HYDROGEN AND METHANE

If your doctor tells you to get a test for just hydrogen, you should insist on testing for methane (and also consider switching specialists!). The bacteria in your gut feed off of carbohydrates and produce hydrogen as a byproduct. However, 8–27% of people do not have detectable levels of hydrogen production in their guts from bacteria. Instead, they produce methane. This is because our guts also contain *archaea,* which are similar to bacteria but in a different kingdom of organisms. Archaea feed off of hydrogen and produce methane gas as a byproduct. So, a bacterial overgrowth could cause increases in hydrogen, methane, or both. We will get into this more in the next chapter which addresses the difference between Hydrogen and Methane SIBO.

Further, certain types of bacteria in the gut produce methane instead of hydrogen. Some of these include: *Staphylococcus aureus, Streptococcus viridans,* Enterococci, Serratia and Pseudomonas species. If you were to test just for hydrogen, you could miss overgrowths of these bacteria and get a false negative.[54]

3-HOUR LACTULOSE TEST IS THE GOLD STANDARD

The 3-Hour Lactulose breath test is considered the Gold Standard for diagnosing SIBO. You may see some laboratories offering shorter tests, such as 60 minutes. These tests are NOT as reliable! It takes time for hydrogen and methane to travel through the gastrointestinal tract, into the blood, and out the lungs into our breath. For this reason, don't waste your time and money on any test but a 3-hour test.[56]

I recommend both Quintron Labs and Commonwealth Labs for SIBO breath testing. They both offer the 3-Hour Lactulose test. The test must be requested by a doctor.

⁸ Methane vs. Hydrogen SIBO

KEY POINTS ABOUT THE TWO TYPES OF SIBO

- SIBO can be methane-producing, hydrogen-producing, or both
- Bacteria produces hydrogen
- Archaea produces methane
- Hydrogen SIBO usually causes diarrhea
- Methane SIBO usually causes constipation
- Breath tests for SIBO will measure levels of methane and hydrogen

When you take a breath test for SIBO, first your baseline hydrogen and methane levels are tested. Then you will take a sugary substance (lactulose) and have your levels tested again.

If your hydrogen levels are high, then you may have Hydrogen-dominant SIBO. If your methane levels are high, then you may have Methane-dominant SIBO. A diagnosis of Hydrogen SIBO or Methane SIBO doesn't mean you only have that type of gas present. You can have both types of gases, just one is more dominant than the other.

*Note I say "may have SIBO" because high breath test levels can indicate other problems as well, not just SIBO.

WHAT'S THE DIFFERENCE BETWEEN HYDROGEN AND METHANE SIBO?

In a healthy gut, food is broken down and absorbed into the blood through the small intestinal wall. With SIBO, there is too much bacteria in your small intestines, and/or the wrong type of bacteria. Bacteria causes unabsorbed carbohydrates in food to ferment before they can break down. The process of fermentation creates hydrogen gas as a byproduct. So, if you have too much bacteria in your small intestines, then you will have high levels of hydrogen—hence the hydrogen breath test for SIBO.

But things aren't that simple. Your small intestines can also contain *archaea*. Archaea feed off of hydrogen. They produce methane as a byproduct. This helps reduce the levels of hydrogen in the body. This is why you can have a negative hydrogen test and still have SIBO.[61]

WHAT ARE ARCHAEA?

Archaea are single celled organisms which lack a nucleus. They are actually pretty cool in that they've been found in virtually all places where anaerobic degradation of organic compounds occurs. They've even been found in the extreme heat of ocean floor vents! Up until recently, archaea were considered a bacteria. However, they are a completely different kingdom than bacteria.[62]

When you eat fiber, the bacteria in your gut start to ferment it. The fermentation produces hydrogen. What do archaea feed off of? Hydrogen! When the archaea consume the hydrogen, they produce methane as a byproduct. In this sense, archaea help reduce the amount of hydrogen gas in our colon—but the methane can have its own negative effects.

A compound which creates methane in the body is called a methanogen. The process of forming methane is called methanogenesis. Some animals rely on methogen-forming archaea. One example is cows which produce a huge amount of methane because of all the bacteria in their stomach which ferment grass. The archaea love the hydrogen from all the fermentation going on. They proliferate and produce methane, which comes out as flatulence. Methane is actually very flammable—don't get any ideas :)

This is a very simplified description of methane production in our bodies, and there are many more pathways involved with methane metabolism. However, for the sake of understanding SIBO, this should be enough.

Interestingly, we don't start producing methane until we are about 3 years old. And not everyone produces methane. Depending on which study you go by, about 33% to 72% of adults produce methane.[62]

BACTERIA → **HYDROGEN** → **ARCHAEA** → **METHANE**
OVERGROWTH   GAS   GAS

PROBLEMS CAUSED BY METHANE

For a long time, people thought that methane was a completely harmless substance in the body—other than causing flatulence and a bit of bloating. However, research is starting to show that high levels of methane may be linked to certain health issues. The main problem caused by methane is constipation (though constipation can be caused by numerous other things).

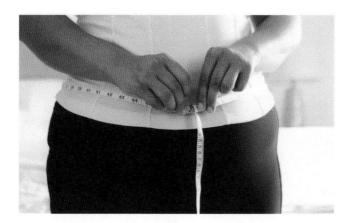

Because methanogens cause a higher production and absorption of short-chain fatty acids, they are also linked to obesity.[63]

Hear that? Methane is linked to obesity. In one study, mice were given a methane-producing archaea and it caused an increase in body fat. In human studies, it was shown that subjects with higher methane levels in their breath tests had higher BMIs.[64]

When it comes to methane and digestive disorders like SIBO, there still isn't much research. However, evidence shows a strong link between methane-producing archaea and SIBO.

As Chris Kresser points out, methane-producing archaea is present in 45% of people with SIBO. Not only that, but the amount of methane produced by people with SIBO is higher.[65]

Is it the archaea themselves which are the cause of the problem? Or are the archaea thriving because they have so much hydrogen to consume because of a bacterial overgrowth? We still need further research to answer these questions, but the answer is probably that *both* too much bacteria and archaea cause problems. That is why experts like Chris Kresser recommend taking steps to eliminate both bacteria and archaea from the small intestine for treating SIBO.

HOW THIS AFFECTS TREATMENT OF SIBO

As a patient, you probably don't need to know about all the scientific differences between archaea and bacteria and how they produce hydrogen and methane. However, it is good to know why your doctor is testing for hydrogen and methane (if your doctor orders only a hydrogen test, insist on getting a methane test too! If the archaea is eating up all the hydrogen, you will have a false negative with the hydrogen test!!!). It is also important to understand that each type of SIBO can have different symptoms.

Here is a picture of my first SIBO breath test. You can see that methane levels are high, not hydrogen—which is a good example of why it is so important to test for *both* hydrogen and methane!

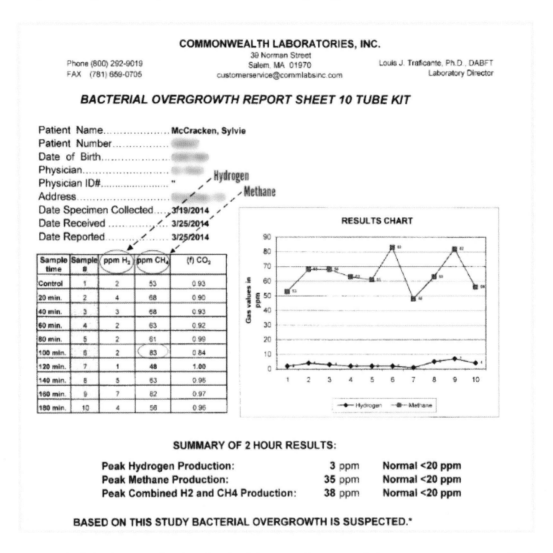

Methane is strongly linked to constipation. So, the following is usually true of the symptoms of SIBO:

- Constipation = methane SIBO

- Diarrhea = hydrogen SIBO

Because of these symptoms, you will often hear the terms SIBO-C (for constipation) and SIBO-D (for diarrhea).

This chart which was published in the journal *Nature*[62] shows the prevalence of constipation and diarrhea in patients with high levels of hydrogen, methane, and both. H_2 = hydrogen. CH_4 = Methane.

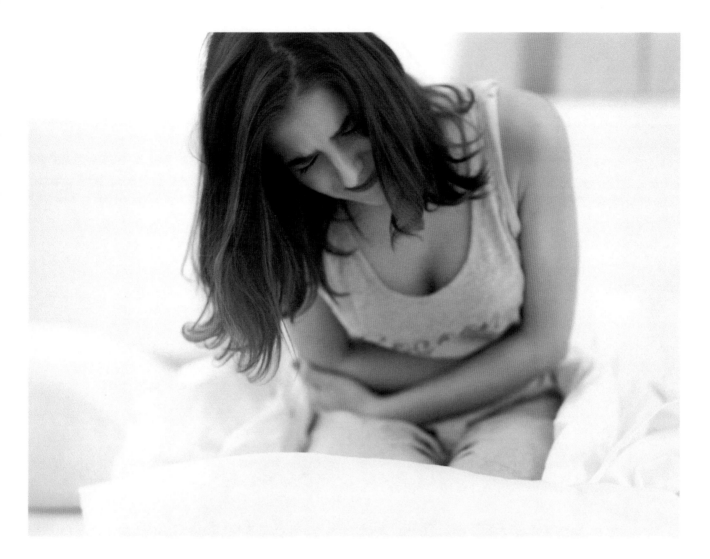

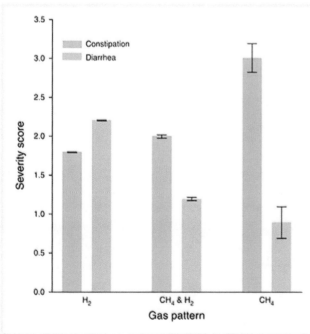

You also need to know that **the treatment for SIBO is different depending on whether it is methane or hydrogen producing.** Most of the archaea which produce methane are somewhat resistant to the antibiotics used to treat SIBO. So, if your problems are caused by archaea overgrowth, then taking those antibiotics aren't likely going to cure your SIBO, even if you take multiple rounds. Methane SIBO is definitely the most difficult to treat because of archaea's resistance to antibiotics.

Actually, antibiotics alone aren't likely to cure any type of SIBO. Sure, if you take enough rounds of antibiotics, you will kill off the bacteria. But antibiotics don't fix the root problem which allowed bacteria to proliferate in the first place, so the SIBO is just likely to come back (hence the high recurrence rate for SIBO). To beat SIBO for good, you need to take comprehensive steps including antibiotics, diet, and lifestyle changes.

⁹ Treating SIBO

HERE IS WHERE WE ARE GOING TO GET INTO THE STEPS YOU NEED TO TAKE TO BEAT SIBO *FOR GOOD*. YOU'LL NOTE THAT I CONSTANTLY SAY "FOR GOOD" WHEN TALKING ABOUT BEATING SIBO. THAT IS BECAUSE SIBO HAS AN INCREDIBLY HIGH RECURRENCE RATE. I WANT TO EMPHASIZE THE FACT THAT IT PROBABLY WON'T BE ENOUGH TO JUST GULP DOWN SOME ANTIBIOTICS TO KILL OFF THE BACTERIA OVERGROWTH. YOU'VE GOT TO TREAT THE ROOT PROBLEMS WHICH ALLOWED OVERGROWTH TO HAPPEN IN THE FIRST PLACE.

Treating SIBO has been a very frustrating but educational process for me. Here is what I did:

- **Round 1:** Antibiotics for two weeks—didn't get rid of the overgrowth, might have made it worse!

- **Round 2:** Vivonex Elemental Diet for 17.5 days followed by prokinetics—didn't get rid of overgrowth but made great progress.

- **Round 3:** Homemade Elemental Diet for 14 days + Herbal Antibiotics followed by prokinetics—negative SIBO results!

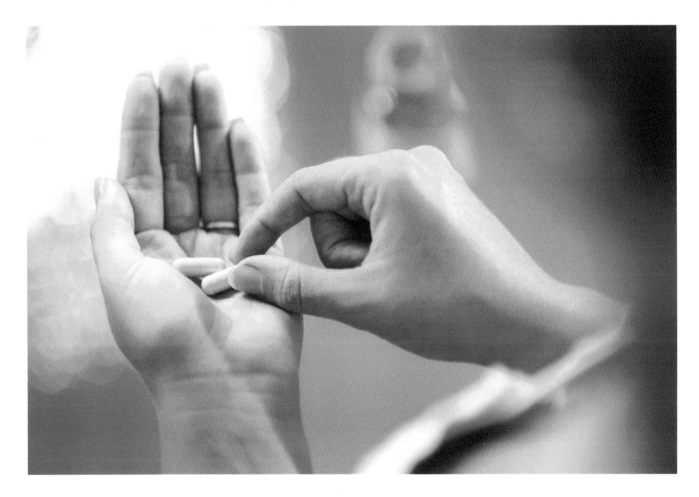

The good news is you likely won't have to go through all of this to cure your SIBO and you can learn from my experiences with each of the treatments. I had a pretty severe case of methane-dominant SIBO, which is the hardest to treat. The initial course of antibiotics didn't come close to getting rid of the SIBO. I was later told that I probably would have likely had to take 4 courses of antibiotics (8 weeks) to beat it and even then they may not have worked, not to mention my body probably wouldn't have been very happy about that. Since antibiotics are ironically also one of the causes of SIBO, and they can have side effects, I didn't want to rely on them again. I decided to go hardcore and tackle it with Elemental Diet, which is the most aggressive treatment option out there. It's the fastest but also the most difficult, no doubt. You can imagine my frustration when even 17.5 days of this didn't completely get rid of the SIBO.

On round 3, I went even more hardcore and attacked SIBO with everything I had: herbal antibiotics, a prokinetic to keep things moving along through the GI tract, and the Elemental Diet. After treatment, I kept taking the prokinetic and did my best to follow the SIBO Diet (though I admittedly slipped up a bit). This is what finally did the trick although I know the first round of elemental also helped set this up for success. I got a negative breath test result which diagnosed me as SIBO free.

Right now, and for the next several months I will be focusing on making sure SIBO doesn't ever come back (since recurrence rates are high). That means taking prokinetics, following the SIBO diet, and getting stress out of my life. So far, so good! Since my SIBO journey will be an ongoing process, and I know many of you would like to hear about any updates or new recommendations that might come up after finalizing this book, feel free to bookmark the resource page where I'll be sure to link any new articles, resources, or updates from me in months and years to come until I'm able to release an updated edition of the book: SIBO resource page www.hollywoodhomestead.com/sibo-solution-resources/

If I had to do it again? I would have done a homemade elemental for three weeks. During the first two weeks of elemental, I would have taken herbal antibiotics. During and after the treatment, I would have taken a prokinetic to keep things moving along. That would have been the fastest, cheapest, and least grueling way to get rid of the overgrowth.

Though treating SIBO has been frustrating, it has also been educational. In the upcoming chapters, I will share with you what I've learned so you can take treatment into your own hands and finally beat this disease for good.

"Treating SIBO is a unique process that requires fine-tuning.

Sylvie personally battled a severe case of SIBO and kicked it to the curb and wants to help you do the same with this incredible guide she's put together.

The SIBO Solution is a must have resource for those treating SIBO.

If you're seeking to understand the complexities of SIBO, eliminate it, and most importantly, make sure it never comes back, you need to get your hands on The SIBO solution."

— **JORDAN REASONER AND STEVE WRIGHT**
SCDLIFESTYLE.COM

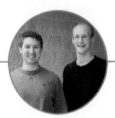

¹⁰ Antibiotics for SIBO

SIBO IS CAUSED BY AN OVERGROWTH OF BACTERIA IN YOUR SMALL INTESTINE, SO IT WOULD MAKE SENSE TO TREAT IT WITH ANTIBIOTICS—RIGHT? WHILE ANTIBIOTICS MAY BE AN INTEGRAL PART OF THE SIBO TREATMENT PROCESS, ANTIBIOTICS ALONE RARELY CURE SIBO IN THE LONG TERM. HERE WE WILL TALK ABOUT WHICH ANTIBIOTICS CAN BE USED FOR TREATING SIBO AND WHY YOU SHOULDN'T RELY SOLELY ON THEM TO OVERCOME SIBO.

WHAT ANTIBIOTICS ARE USED FOR TREATING SIBO?

There are two antibiotics which are mainly used for treating SIBO: Rifaximin (generic: Xifaxan) and Neomycin (added in addition to Rifaximin in the case of methane-dominant SIBO). The reason these are chosen is because they are *non-systemic,* meaning they mostly don't get absorbed into the bloodstream and instead stay in the intestines, allowing them to kill bacteria residing in the intestines and not elsewhere. Less frequently, the systemic antibiotic (meaning it *does* get into your blood and circulate through your body) Metronidazole is prescribed.[66] Generally, doctors will prescribe these antibiotics for 10 to 14 day courses.[67] These antibiotics are expensive (about $1000 for a 14 day course of Rifaximin in the US) and often not covered by insurance.

At siboinfo.com, Dr. Siebecker (a leading expert on SIBO) gives these as some examples of SIBO dosage options. Keep in mind that there aren't any established protocols for SIBO antibiotic dosages, so your doctor may prescribe something different:[66]

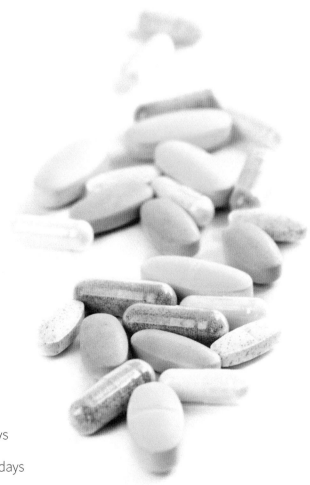

- Rifaximin 1600mg daily × 10 days

- Rifaximin 1200mg daily × 14 days

- Rifaximin 1600mg daily + Neomycin 1000mg daily × 10 days

- Rifaximin 1600mg daily + Metronidazole 750mg daily × 10 days

Oftentimes, a single round with one of these antibiotics doesn't cure SIBO, especially in severe cases.[1] When the first course doesn't work, doctors will often prescribe another antibiotic or add another antibiotic to the treatment for another course. For me, one 14 day course of Rifaximin + Neomycin didn't even come close to eradicating SIBO. Although I didn't retest immediately after so I can't tell you how much progress it did make or how fast recurrence was, I can tell you my symptoms were not relieved and over the following months continued to get worse. I later learned that based on my severe case it likely would have taken at least FOUR rounds! If I'd known that, I wouldn't even have done the first round, saving me time, money (not only on treatment but testing and doctors visits) and the anguish associated with all of that.

But Don't Antibiotics *Cause* SIBO?

It is ironic that antibiotics are used to treat SIBO, because antibiotics are also one of the main causes of SIBO.

Antibiotics can't tell the difference between the "healthy" bacteria in your body and the "harmful" bacteria. They also can't determine healthy levels of bacteria (remember, SIBO can sometimes be caused by too much of the healthy bacteria which *should* be in your gut!). When you take an antibiotic, whether for SIBO or another condition, it will indiscriminately kill off *all* bacteria—including the good guys.

The good bacteria in our guts have many roles, including keeping the "bad guys" in check. Without enough good guys, the bad guys can quickly get out of control. So, those antibiotics for SIBO might *temporarily* get rid of the harmful bacteria, but it will probably just come back since you also killed off the good guys too! Hence why SIBO has such a high recurrence rate.

The (In)Effectiveness of Antibiotics for Treating SIBO

Depending on which reports you go by, antibiotics are 40% to 91% effective in treating SIBO.[66, 67]

However, if we look at the long-term effectiveness of antibiotics for treating SIBO, the results are poor. ***Studies show that recurrence occurs in almost HALF of all patients within one year!***[1]

Considering that antibiotics kill off the healthy bacteria in your gut, the high recurrence rate of SIBO after antibiotic treatment shouldn't be surprising. More importantly, **antibiotics do not address the underlying conditions which caused bacteria overgrowth in the first place.** This is why it is so important to take a comprehensive approach to SIBO treatment which includes taking a prokinetic (which we talk about later in chapter 13), and making changes to your diet and lifestyle. You can't just expect that a hardcore round of antibiotics is going to solve your problems! There is no magic pill for SIBO and that includes antibiotics.

> ***You must wait 14 days after finishing a round of antibiotics (even herbal antibiotics) before retesting. This is critical for the accuracy of test! However, don't wait more than 16 days to retest; you want to retest before regrowth of bacteria (recurrence) has time to occur.**

Remember: these antibiotics require a prescription and I'm not a doctor. In the US, these antibiotics are often costly, even with insurance. Since I'm uninsured I bought them (legally) from an online pharmacy in Canada for $\frac{1}{10}$th the cost. Going that route will still require you to have a prescription and might require some patience on the shipping front.

¹¹ Herbal Antibiotics for SIBO

THERE IS NO DENYING THAT ANTIBIOTICS ARE ONE OF THE MOST BENEFICIAL MEDICAL INNOVATIONS OF MODERN HISTORY. THEY HAVE HELPED ERADICATE MANY COMMUNICABLE DISEASES AND SAVED COUNTLESS LIVES. BUT ANTIBIOTICS HAVE ALSO BROUGHT WITH THEM A NUMBER OF UNFORESEEN PROBLEMS AND HEALTH RISKS.

Before we go any further, I want to say that I'm not anti doctor nor anti traditional medicine, but each has its time and a place. Antibiotics are often over pre-scribed and shouldn't be our default first choice for treating everything. For numerous reasons, many peo-ple are turning to herbal antibiotics for treating SIBO.

WHAT IS AN ANTIBIOTIC?

According to MedicineNet.com, an antibiotic is:

A drug used to treat bacterial infections. Originally, an antibiotic was a substance produced by one microorgan-ism that selectively inhibits the growth of another. Syn-thetic antibiotics, usually chemically related to natural antibiotics, have since been produced that accomplish comparable tasks.

As humans, we have been using natural antibiotics for centuries, even before we knew what bacteria was. For example, garlic has been used since at least 2600BC for its healing properties. Today, we now know that garlic has natural antibacterial properties.

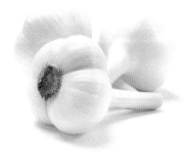

WHY CHOOSE HERBAL ANTIBIOTICS FOR TREATING SIBO?

There are already several pharmaceutical antibiotics which are commonly prescribed for SIBO. So why would you choose herbal antibiotics over these? There are three main reasons:

I   Antibiotic resistance

II Fewer potential side effects

III Herbal antibiotics may be more effective

1. Herbs Don't Cause Antibiotic Resistance

In 1929, Alexander Fleming discovered penicillin and changed modern medicine completely. Doctors were convinced that antibiotics would cure all bacterial dis-eases. In 1963, the Australian physician and Nobel Prize winner Sir Macfarlane Burnet even said that by the end of the 20th century humanity would see the "virtual elimina-tion of infectious disease as a significant factor in societal life." In 1970, the Surgeon General William Stewart said that antibiotics would soon "close the book on infectious diseases." They couldn't have been more wrong!

What they didn't realize was that bacteria are capable of adapting to antibiotics and becoming resistant to them. This is a VERY serious problem, and one which shouldn't be taken lightly. Thanks to antibiotic resistance, diseases which were once treatable—such as tuberculosis—are now often fatal. We may soon see the re-emergence of diseases like typhoid, diphtheria, and many others.[68]

Keep in mind that antibiotics are not always effective in treating SIBO. Even when the first round of antibiotics works, the SIBO often comes back after just a short time. As researchers point out in an article in *Gastroenterology,*[69] SIBO patients often require multiple rounds or continuous courses of antibiotic therapy. To prevent resistance, they recommend rotating antibiotic regimens to prevent resistance.

Herbal antibiotics work on multiple levels in the body, so resistance is less likely to occur. Further, by using herbal remedies instead of turning to pharmaceuticals every time you get sick, you slow the spread of antibiotic resistance.[70, 71]

2. Fewer Side effects with Herbal Antibiotics for SIBO

There are three main drugs which are used for treating SIBO: Rifaximin, Neomycin, and Metronidazole. Each of these has some pretty nasty potential side effects. I've listed some of them below—but bear in mind that these are just *some* of the potential side effects.

Drug	Common Side Effect	Less Common Side Effect
Rifaximin	Bloating, Gas, Stomach pain, Nausea, Constipation, Headache, Dizziness, Feeling tired, Trouble sleeping	Muscle spasms, Fainting, Ulcers in the mouth, Chest pain
Neomycin	Irritation in mouth or rectal area, Nausea and Vomiting	Dizziness, Low of hearing, Ringing sound in ears, Skin rash
Metronidazole	Feeling agitated, Back pain, Confusion, Vomiting, Weakness and Unsteadiness, Depression	Blood in stools, Body aches and pains, Severe stomach pain, Nasal congestion, Couching, Bleeding gums

As if dealing with SIBO symptoms isn't bad enough, you've also got to worry about antibiotic side effects!

With herbal antibiotics, there is still a risk of side effects. However, the side effects generally aren't going to be as severe as with prescription antibiotics.[70]

One point worth mentioning is that **even herbal antibiotics can kill off good bacteria**. So, even you use herbal antibiotics instead of prescription ones, *you still must make diet and lifestyle changes to help restore gut symbiosis.*

3. Herbal Antibiotics Are Effective

Need another reason to choose herbal antibiotics for SIBO? How about the fact that they may be *more effective* in treating SIBO than prescription antibiotics!

Now, bear in mind that there have been really few studies on *pharmaceutical* antibiotics for SIBO. There have been even fewer for herbal antibiotics for SIBO. In fact, there are only two (yes, TWO!) studies to date which look at how herbal antibiotics can treat SIBO. And one of these studies was on just one person![72]

However, the lack of research doesn't mean that herbal antibiotics aren't a good solution. In the larger study, which was published in the journal *Global Advances in Health and Medicine*[73], the results are pretty impressive. They took 104 people who had been diagnosed with SIBO through lactulose breath testing. Of these, 37 of the patients were treated with herbal antibiotics and the remaining were given Rifaximin.

The results? 46% of the patients who took herbal antibiotics had a negative breath test upon follow-up, compared to just 34% of the Rifaximin users. The researchers concluded that herbal therapies are "at least as effective as Rifaximin for resolution of SIBO."

Doctor Siebecker, who is a leading expert on treating SIBO, says that she and her associates have regularly used herbal antibiotics for SIBO since 2011 and "have consistently found them to be as effective as pharmaceutical antibiotics in relieving symptoms and reducing gas levels on breath testing."[72]

What Makes Herbal Antibiotics So Effective?

Why would a natural substance be more effective than the prescription drugs which scientists worked for years to develop? The book *Herbal Antibiotics* by Stephan Harrod Buhner describes it well (find the book on our resource page at www.hollywoodhomestead.com/sibo-solution-resources/). He talks about how pharmaceutical antibiotics are isolated chemicals—meaning they are one chemical. Because they are only one thing, it is easier for bacteria to adapt to them and develop a resistance.

By contrast, herbs are made up of many compounds. For example, garlic (which is one of the best known natural antibiotics) contains *dozens* of compounds. All of these compounds work together and can attack bacteria on multiple levels. It is much harder for bacteria to adapt to herbal antibiotics because of how complex the herbs' structures are.[70]

Even the individual compounds in herbs can work in complex ways. Allicin, which is one of the main antibacterial compounds found in garlic, is a particularly good example of the complexity of herbal antibiotics. Interestingly, allicin isn't present in undamaged garlic. But, when the garlic becomes damaged, a chemical reaction occurs and allicin is produced to protect the plant from disease and other damage (that is why garlic becomes pungent once you cut it open). Once in the body, allicin undergoes a redox-reaction with proteins, which is thought to be the source of its biological activity.[74]

*Allicin does not contain the FODMAPs part of garlic (which means it won't ferment), so it is okay to take for SIBO.

Here is some food for thought. Animals can move, and this allows them to come up with evolutionary survival mechanisms like being able to run fast or have sharp claws to fight predators. Plants don't have the ability to move, so they've had to come up with other ways of protecting themselves. They've evolved chemical structures to protect themselves—like how poison ivy will make you itch or kale tastes bitter so animals won't want to eat it. These mechanisms have been perfected in *millions* of years of evolution (definitely longer than we've been creating chemicals in labs!).

With a bit of research, we could utilize these natural plant compounds for our own benefit. Consider the fact that about 40% of all prescription medicines are plant-derived. About 25% of these come from the rainforest, and we've only tested fewer than 1% of all the tropical trees and plants in the rainforest![74, 75]

The bottom line? Plants are pretty amazing and their healing powers shouldn't be underestimated.

Which Herbal Antibiotics Treat SIBO?

Unfortunately, there hasn't been much research into herbal antibiotics, and even less research about herbal antibiotics specifically for treating SIBO (it seems that drug companies would rather fund research for expensive chemical pharmaceuticals than cheap, natural remedies!).

Here is the herbal antibiotic regimen I used for treating SIBO:

- **Allimed (Allicin) 450mg:** Allicin is a component of garlic. Take 1–2 caps 3× per day for a total of 14 days (start with 1 cap 3× per day and on day 3 increase to 2 caps 3× per day). It is important that you take 450mg! Find out where to buy it on our resource page here: www.hollywoodhomestead.com/sibo-solution-resources/. You will need 2 bottles for a 14 day course.

- **Berberine Complex:** Berberine is a compound found in Oregon grape, barberry, goldenseal, and other herbs. Take 2–3 caps 3× per day for a total of 14 days (start with 2 caps 3× per day and on day 3 increase to 3 caps 3× per day; can cause headaches). Find out where to buy it on our resource page here: www.hollywoodhomestead.com/sibo-solution-resources/. You will need to buy 2 bottles for a 14 day course.

Neem Plus: Neem is a tropical evergreen tree. Take 1 cap 3× per day for a total of 14 days. Find out where to buy it on our resource page here: www.hollywoodhomestead.com/sibo-solution-resources/. You will need 1 bottle for a 14 day course.

I took all 3 of these herbal antibiotics for a 14 day course. Many people take herbal antibiotics for SIBO even longer though—such as 1 month courses. I took these herbal antibiotics *while I was doing the elemental diet*. You don't have to do elemental though. In fact, many people do either/or.

There are two schools of thought about using antibiotics or herbal antibiotics while on the elemental diet (which starves the bacteria). Some doctors say you need to feed the bacteria while taking antibiotics so they're active while you kill them instead of lying dormant while they're dying off on elemental. I can tell you that doing both elemental and herbal simultaneously worked for me.

I ALSO TOOK:

Interfase Plus (Klaire Labs): This is a biofilm disruptor. It is unclear how much it actually helps, but it certainly doesn't hurt and I was at the "let's toss the kitchen sink at this" approach. Take 2 caps 3× per day. If doing elemental, take away from the elemental formula as much as possible. Find out where to buy it on our resource page here: www.hollywoodhomestead.com/sibo-solution-resources/. You will need 1 bottle for a 14 day course.

MotilPro (Pure Encapsulations): This one is for the long term. It's a prokinetic. It's mostly ginger and does cause a bit of burning so some dislike it but I've found it effective. Take with lots of water to minimize that burning sensation in the esophagus. Take 3 caps before bed and 3 caps 1–2 times a day between meals. Find out where to buy it on our

resource page here: www.hollywoodhomestead.com/sibo-solution-resources/. Go ahead and buy 2 bottles, 1 for the herbal antibiotics course and another bottle for post-treatment.

*While I totally understand why someone would choose herbal antibiotics over prescription antibiotics, it is important to note that herbal antibiotics courses are often much longer. It is like using a handgun instead of a grenade :)

IMPORTANT NOTES ABOUT HERBAL ANTIBIOTICS FOR SIBO

Whether you are taking herbal or pharmaceutical antibiotics for SIBO, you must wait 14 days after finishing a round before retesting. This is critical for the accuracy of test! However, don't wait more than 16 days to retest; you want to retest before regrowth of bacteria (recurrence) has time to occur.

After finishing with herbal or pharmaceutical antibiotics, you will need to take a prokinetic agent (I took MotilPro during the herbal antibiotics course and added 2 more prokinetics post-treatment). You can start with the prokinetic immediately after antibiotics, even before you've retested. Read more about prokinetics in chapter 13 about Motility.

Remember, herbal antibiotics may be a better alternative to pharmaceutical antibiotics—but even these aren't the sole solution to treating SIBO. To get rid of SIBO *and keep it away*, you've got to treat the underlying issues which caused the bacterial overgrowth in the first place. That means making changes to your diet and life.

> "I used the protocol outlined in the book and it worked beautifully. Having the knowledge that I could bypass the antibiotic protocol my doctor wanted to prescribe was priceless. Thank you for the SIBO Solution!"
>
> — LINDA

¹² Elemental Diet

AFTER HAVING LIMITED SUCCESS WITH TRADITIONAL ANTIBIOTICS, I DECIDED TO TAKE THE TREATMENT TO A WHOLE 'NOTHER LEVEL. ONE IMPORTANT STEP THAT I DID TO TREAT MY SEVERE CASE OF SIBO WAS DO AN ELEMENTAL DIET.

WHAT IS AN ELEMENTAL DIET?

An elemental diet, also often called a bowel reset diet, isn't actually a diet in the traditional sense at all. It is a short-term protocol in which you *eat nothing*. The goal of elemental is to starve off the bacteria in your small intestine. To prevent your body from starving, you take a special liquid formula (formulated for tube feeding patients) which contains predigested nutrients. The nutrients are easily assimilated into the body so bacteria can't feed off of them and proliferate. Elemental diets are also often used to treat Crohn's Disease, a condition in which the gastrointestinal tract is severely inflamed. By taking the liquid Elemental Diet instead of eating, the gut is able to start healing.

HOW DOES AN ELEMENTAL DIET TREAT SIBO?

Remember that bacteria are living things. Like all living things, bacteria have to eat something. The bacteria in our small intestines primarily live off of certain carbohydrates that we eat. When you eat these fermentable sugars, you aren't just feeding yourself but the bacteria too!

This doesn't mean you shouldn't ever eat carbs. Remember, it is normal and healthy to have some level of bacteria in our guts. The problem occurs when you've got too many of certain carbs in your gut. The bacteria have a smorgasbord and start to proliferate out of control. This leads to SIBO, which in turn can lead to other serious problems like leaky gut. Bear in mind that some carbs are a lot worse than others, and there are a lot of reasons why you might have excess carbs in your small intestine.

When you are on an Elemental Diet, you eat *nothing*. Instead, you take a liquid formula which contains predigested nutrients so they are absorbed into your bloodstream quickly and the bacteria can't use them for food. So, the bacteria have nothing to feed off of and die off.

DOES IT WORK?

An elemental diet is no doubt a hardcore way to deal with SIBO—but it is an effective one. In one study, 93 subjects with IBS and SIBO (diagnosed with a high lactulose breath test) were put on an elemental diet. After 15 days, 80% of them had negative breath tests.[76] According to RD Kelsey Marksteiner, elemental diet has a cure rate of 80–85% for SIBO.[77] Compare this to the cure rate of antibiotics for SIBO (which is as low as 40%), and the elemental diet is definitely worth considering, especially in severe cases.

Because your gut is able to rest and heal itself while on the elemental diet, it might help cure some of the underlying causes of SIBO and thus reduce recurrence rate. However, there aren't any studies (that I am aware of at least) which show what the SIBO recurrence rate is for elemental vs. other forms of treatment.

Pros and Cons of the Elemental Diet

The main pro of an elemental diet for treating SIBO is that it is a fast and effective treatment which doesn't require a prescription. However, this effectiveness doesn't come without drawbacks. The main one is that doing an elemental diet is NOT at all a pleasant experience! You can't have any solid food and those powered elemental formulas aren't exactly the best tasting thing. Elemental diets usually should last around 2 or 3 weeks to be effective, so you've got to be able to tough it out that long.

Another drawback of the elemental diet is that it can be pricey. Readymade store bought elemental formulas for SIBO cost about $1000 for 2 weeks. You can save money by making your own elemental formulas. However, even homemade elemental formulas are still going to be a bit pricy because you've got to purchase all of the nutrients individually. Expect to pay about $300–$400 for 2 weeks.

Should You Do Elemental?

Even though the elemental diet has a higher cure rate than traditional antibiotics, it is understandable that most people wouldn't want to turn to it as a first-choice treatment option. Doing elemental is not at all a pleasant experience, and you will have to make some serious lifestyle changes while doing it.

I would recommend doing elemental for SIBO under these circumstances:

- Your SIBO case is severe (methane and/or hydrogen numbers over 80 at any point in the 3 hour test)

- You've tried traditional or herbal antibiotics for SIBO but haven't had much success

- You are ready for the extreme measure of going without food (you've got to do it 2–3 weeks for it to be effective)

- Losing a few pounds would not be detrimental to your health (i.e. if you're already underweight, you may want to rethink it)

- You have SIBO along with another gut disease where severe inflammation is in place, such as Crohn's or IBS

- You're so very over it and ready to just be done with SIBO once and for all

Elemental Diet Options

You've got two options when it comes to the elemental diet for SIBO: you can buy a readymade formula (Vivonex Plus) or do a homemade formula. I did both of these options (Vivonex the first round, and homemade the second). Overall, I like homemade better. It was easier to mix up than I anticipated and I just mixed it once a day and portioned out 3 jars in the fridge.

Let's talk about each of the elemental diet options so you can decide if either is right for you.

Vivonex Plus:

It is definitely pricey at about $1000 for two weeks, but it's the easiest. You just add water and take it. This formula has also actually been studied and proven effective. Find out where to buy Vivonex on our resource page here: www.hollywoodhomestead.com/sibo-solution-resources/. You will need to buy enough for about 6 packets per day. A drawback with the Vivonex Plus option is that it does contain some not-ideal ingredients (mainly corn derived) which are actually contraindicated in SIBO (yes, this means it could still feed the bacteria a tiny bit, slowing down the die-off). It is high carbohydrate /low fat, so this also won't be ideal for everyone.[78]

Another point worth mentioning about Vivonex is that *it tastes horrible*. The smell alone is enough to make you gag. It's meant to be a tube feeding formula so I guess they never took smell and flavor into account when formulating it. I could not get past 2–3 sips of it without gagging. The only way I could get it down was by adding Crystal Light. Yes, I know the ingredients in

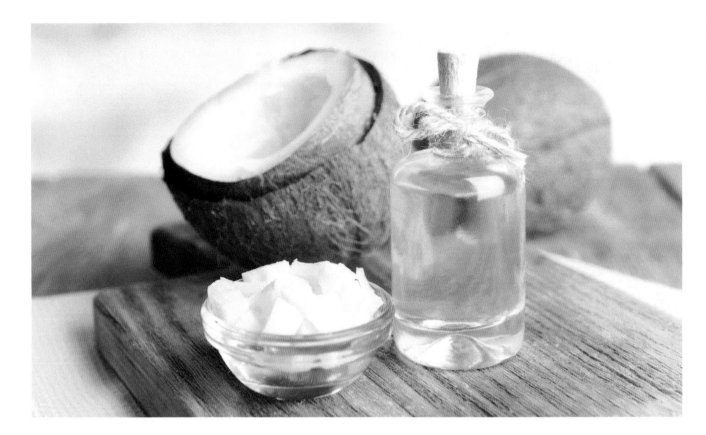

Crystal Light are terrible (soy, dyes, artificial sweeteners, etc.), but it was the best solution I found and recommended by my doctor, and I had to prioritize starving the bacteria for this short treatment time. That said, because I added the Crystal Light most of the time I couldn't tell if a headache or other symptom was a die off reaction or just a reaction to the daily dosing of soy and artificial dyes which my body isn't used to. I decided it didn't matter and plowed ahead for 17.5 days.

HOMEMADE ELEMENTAL FORMULA:

If you want to save money, gag a little less and consume ingredients that are slightly closer to real food, this is the way to go. Expect to pay about $300–$400 for 2 weeks. The ingredients are a lot cleaner since you're able to choose each one individually. Another plus of going with the homemade route is that you will be able to adjust the amount of carbs and fats a bit to your needs. Bear in mind that you will have to buy each ingredient separately and mix them together each day. The oil doesn't mix well so I ended up sipping this separately, which isn't exactly tasty.

Recipes for Homemade Elemental Formula

These recipes come from Dr. Siebecker (reprinted with her permission). There are two options: high fat/low carb and low fat/high carb. I did the high fat option. Make sure to use quality ingredients because this is what you are going to be living off of for the next 2 weeks. You can find out where to buy the ingredients on our resource page here: www.hollywoodhomestead.com/sibo-solution-resources/.

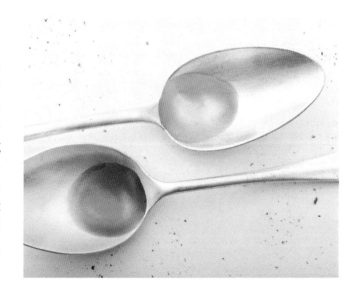

- 2.2 lbs Jo Mar Labs Amino Acids (Original, No-MSM)

- 10 lbs Dextrose

- Half gallon high-quality oil: I used a combo of organic coconut and olive oil. You can also use cod liver oil or macadamia oil. Make sure it is great quality.

- 1 bottle Pure Encapsulations Nutrient 950 Multivitamin

- Unrefined Celtic Sea Salt

- Optional flavorings (such as vanilla) in small amounts per dose

LOW CARB/HIGH FAT OPTION:

These instructions are *per dose/meal*. If you are going to mix everything up at the start/end of the day, then multiply everything by 3 and divide it into 3 cups to put in the fridge.

- **2 Tbsp amino acids (24 grams)**

- **3.5–5 Tbsp dextrose (3.5T = 35g carbs, 5T = 50g carbs)**

- **3–3.5 Tbsp oil (3T = 41g fat, 3.5T = 49g fat)***

- **2 capsules of the multivitamin, emptied out**

- **¼ to ½ tsp salt**

*If using higher dextrose amount, use lower oil amount, or use higher oil amount if using lower dextrose amount.

LOW FAT/HIGH CARB OPTION:

These instructions are *per dose/meal*. If you are going to mix everything up at the start/end of the day, then multiply everything by 3 and divide it into 3 cups to put in the fridge.

- **2 Tbsp + 1 tsp amino acids (28 grams)**

- **⅔ cup dextrose (106g carbs)**

- **1 tsp oil (4.6g fat)**

- **2 capsules of the multivitamin, emptied out**

- **¼ to ½ tsp salt**

Just mix everything together in a blender with water. You can use as much or little water as you want to get a desired thickness. You can add ice too. Never use juice, milk or any other liquid but water to blend the ingredients!

Alternatively, you can take each of the ingredients individually. However, it is probably better to sip it throughout the day, even if it doesn't taste so fabulous. Using small amounts of vanilla extract as flavorings is allowed but honestly I found it made it taste even worse. I think this is because I found it obnoxiously sweet from the dextrose and the vanilla seemed to accentuate that. It was nowhere near as terrible tasting as the Vivonex however.

Find out where to buy each of these ingredients on our resource page here: www.hollywoodhomestead.com/sibo-solution-resources/.

Elemental Diet Dosage

An elemental diet needs to last 2–3 weeks to be effective. With Vivonex Plus, you use 6 packets per day (you can double them up and take 2 packets, 3 times a day or take the 6 packets separately, as you wish), which comes out to 1800 calories per day. With the homemade elemental, the dosage is 3× per day, which comes out to about 2000 calories.

Keep in mind you don't have to take the formula 3× or 6× per day. You really have a lot of flexibility with how you take it and can adjust it to your activity and caloric needs. For example, while doing the Vivonex elemental formula, there were days when I just laid around in bed and rested. I didn't need a full 1800 calories during those days, so I took 5 or sometimes even just 4 drinks per day. Consult with your doc to see what is best for you!

Retesting After Elemental Diet

After completing the Elemental Diet, you need to wait at least 4 days before retesting. This gives things time to settle down—but don't wait more than 2 weeks or you might not get accurate results. The idea is for the test to tell you how effective the treatment was, even if some mild re-feeding happens when you start reintroducing food again.

On my first round, I retested after 4 days. On my second round, I did it at 2 weeks after because it also co-incided with the retesting schedule of the herbal antibiotics I took simultaneously with elemental. (Retesting after antibiotics requires a 2 week waiting period as we discuss in <u>chapter 10</u> on page <u>47</u>).

> "I am so grateful to find your book!
>
> I did not understand anything about SIBO until I read your book — VERY INFORMATIVE! Thank you!"

My Personal Experience with the Elemental Diet

Before doing the first round of elemental diet, I was both excited and scared. Excited at the thought that this would be the quickest way to get results (it was). Scared because I'd heard stories of people not being able to make it past day 4 because they felt so terrible.

Because my case was so severe, I did Elemental for 17.5 days the first round. I hoped the extra days would mean I would never have to do this again. Close, but not quite. The results from that breath test were better, but I still had work to do. So I did another round of Elemental, this time using the homemade formula and for 13.5 days.

Important! I also took herbal antibiotics and a prokinetic while doing the second round of elemental. Read about the importance of prokinetics in <u>chapter 13</u>.

How I Felt While on Elemental Diet

VIVONEX PLUS (ROUND 1):

I started on a Monday (isn't that how diets are supposed to roll? ;) and I was armed with my drinks made up for the following day, plenty of ice in the freezer to pour them over and, aside from loads of movies to watch, an almost blank to-do list. I also started a diary on Evernote to keep track of how I felt.

I was worried when day 4 rolled around since I had heard that days 4–8 were the worst in regards to bacterial die-off. But, for me, it was actually days 8–12 that were the worst, probably because my case was so severe. During those days, I had diarrhea and terrible bloating and cramping. I relied on detox protocols during this time (especially Epsom salt baths and castor oil packs) to help me through.

Symptoms throughout:

I had headaches which started pretty much on day 1. It might not have been related to SIBO but to the corn and soy ingredients which I don't react well to. I also often felt itchy and had lots of phlegm. Again, it could have been the ingredients. My breath was terrible and there was some moderate body odor, which is unusual when I'm eating a clean diet. There was some cramping and insane amounts of burping—even in the middle of the night! The bloating was so bad that I looked like was 6–8 months pregnant depending on the time of day. It was interesting to see this after 10 days of not eating! Clearly, the party in my gut was starting to get disrupted. And one more weird side effect: my teeth started to hurt.

My energy levels were okay for the first few days and then I started to feel lethargic. It could have been the bacterial die-off, but I think inadvertently I wasn't consuming enough calories because I hated the taste of the drinks so much that I was limiting them to just enough to keep me alive. If I had to do Vivonex Plus again, I'd add some high quality oil like olive oil to sip in addition to the drinks since their profile is pretty low fat.

Here is a post from my diary (Day 11):

The brain fog is unreal. My writing looks dyslexic. And I'm not trying to be funny. Simple math in my head seems impossible. And finding words is very difficult. It's like my mom when she's trying to speak English except it happens to me in both languages and at any time of day even after a good night's sleep. It's like the synapses just aren't happening.

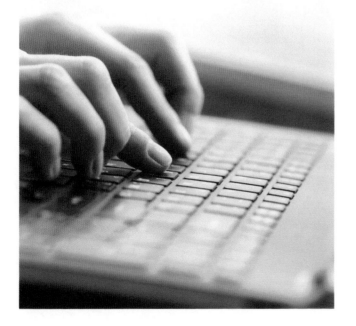

How I Felt After Vivonex:

The truth is I was expecting to feel instantly better the minute I got off elemental. I mean, that's as low as my breath test results would ever be, I wasn't eating anything for pete's sake! But, the truth is, although I felt instantly better just having some real food (albeit sticking to very simple, bland things like ground beef and small amounts of cooked SIBO friendly vegetables), the SIBO symptoms were not immediately completely gone. Both times my body was a bit shocked and confused to be eating again and digestion seemed slow. I was also a bit scared to eat which may seem silly but I'm just trying to be honest.

"The SIBO solution is the resource for anyone struggling from small intestinal bacterial overgrowth. Sylvie has provided a thorough guide to help you navigate the issues, symptoms, and options for understanding and treating the condition. Her holistic approach to dealing with SIBO sheds lights on the complex relationship between our gut and overall health. She provides practical solutions, tons of resources, and up-to-date research. Her personal story and honest portrayal of her own struggles makes her that "been there done that" supportive friend you need to discover solutions you seek."

I highly recommend this book to anyone who has (or wonders if they might have) SIBO.

— **ROBIN KONIE**, THANKYOURBODY.COM

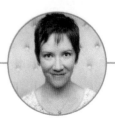

RESULTS:

Original Test Results

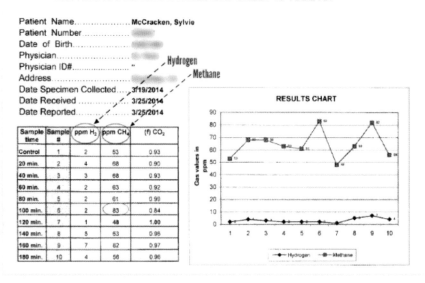

Test Results After Vivonex Elemental for 17.5 days

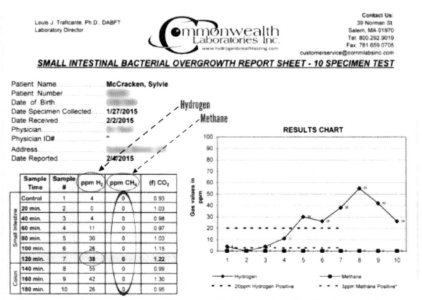

As you can see my methane numbers (which were previously very high) were zero across the board. This is great! But what was surprising was that my hydrogen numbers, previously nominal, had increased enough to still technically be a positive result. I later found out this is actually quite typical. I was on the right track but more work needed to be done.

The second round of elemental was much easier. This is most likely because I had made a ton of progress on the first round so there was less die-off and thus fewer symptoms. However, it was still emotionally tough to feel deprived of food. After that round of elemental was over I noticed that, while again I didn't have life-changing nirvana immediately after finishing, I felt better with each day that passed by. I was more energized and less bloated. It was like the healing was still happening even though I wasn't doing anything for it anymore. Sort of like when you step off a treadmill and your heart is still pounding and sweating for quite a bit longer.

The reason I decided to do a second round of elemental, with the thumbs up from my doctor, is that I felt so close and knew it would take much longer to make progress with something like diet alone. I just wanted to eliminate so I would only need to focus on prevention which is a much easier, yet just as important undertaking.

Results of second round of Elemental—this time homemade:

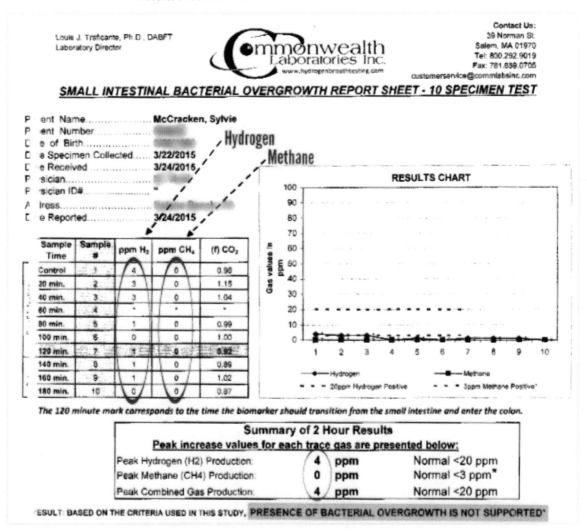

SIBO clear! The results on this one was just about zero.

As you can see this time both hydrogen and methane numbers where down to zero/almost zero. Finally SIBO clear!

The whole experience was a like a flashback to my "dieting" days. Yes, it made me feel deprived at times. An interesting thing though is that I found Elemental easier than those weight loss diets I used to do. For some reason, it was easier to swear off all food completely than the superhuman willpower it takes to have "just one" bite of cake. Gretchen Rubin in her book *Better Than Before* refers to this type of habit former as The Abstainer. You can find the book on our resource page here: www.hollywoodhomestead.com/sibo-solution-resources/.

Elemental also had an unexpected benefit for me. As a mother of three kids aged 4 to 16 and a business owner, I don't get too much down time and I have to manage a lot of things. This was an opportunity to ask my husband and older daughter to pick up some of the slack for a couple of weeks so I could focus on resting. Plus, I hired a housekeeper to help out as well. I didn't deal with cooking or grocery shopping (which would have been torture while not eating!), so this freed up a lot of time which I could use to focus on relaxing and de-stressing. Again, stress is the biggest cause of SIBO! Many of those tasks I didn't take back on after my elemental diet was over ;)

My Best Advice for you during your Elemental Diet:

1. Get Support!

Without the help that I had during both rounds of elemental, I guarantee I wouldn't have made it through it. And I don't just mean help around the house, with the kids, or time off work. I also mean emotional support. The toughest times for me were evenings and weekends, during my family's meal times. I stayed in my bedroom, turned on my essential oil diffuser (the peppermint seemed particularly soothing) so I wouldn't smell the delicious food and/or I took an Epsom salt bath. Having my husband to talk me off the ledge when I could have killed someone for a piece of chicken was incredibly helpful. He offered to bring me tea and took the kids out for dinner a few times so I wouldn't smell food.

2. Get Time Off Work

Ideally take 2 weeks off and make it your full time job to get well. If you have limited time off, try to schedule it to start after day 4 since that's when it starts to get difficult, emotionally and also with die-off symptoms. If necessary, ask your doctor about disability insurance. This condition is no joke.

3. Clothing

Do yourself a favor and forget jeans or anything restrictive in the waist. Yoga pants are your friend. I lived in maxi dresses, yoga pants with long shirts and pajamas.

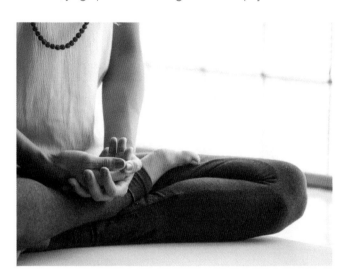

> "I'm on week 3 of the FODMAP diet. Sylvie's book really helped jump start me on this protocol and gave me the motivation to start. After procrastinating for 4 years this was no small deal! I felt that if Sylvie could do it so could I! She lays things out very comprehensively. I especially liked the recipe section because it made me realize that FODMAP can be tasty after all!"
>
> **— Ondina Hatvany**

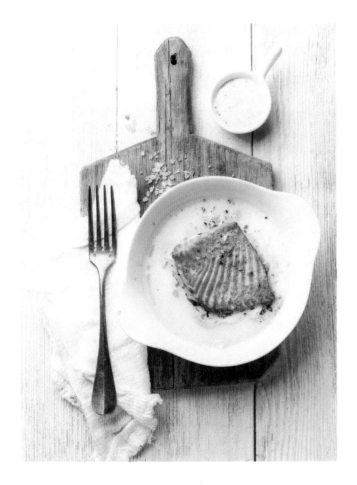

6. THE GROSS FILM ON YOUR TEETH

The elemental diet (especially Vivonex Plus) leaves this weird gross film on your teeth. Brushing with baking soda and a couple drops of Orawellness oil blend was the easiest way to handle this. Also, try oil pulling for the teeth pain. Orawellness is listed on our resource page here: www.hollywoodhomestead.com/sibo-solution-resources/.

7. MAKE THE TIME PASS

During the first round of elemental, I had a pity party for myself and the 17 ½ days seemed like an eternity. During the second round, I tried to keep busy by writing, working, and organizing my files and photos (all mostly from my bed) and the time went by a lot quicker.

If you're in the middle of your elemental diet as you're reading this, just remember time doesn't stand still, although it can sometimes feel that way. You're making progress every single day, getting closer to the end of your treatment, and the end of your SIBO journey. Hang in there. Get a countdown timer app on your phone for when you need the occassional reminder of just how far you've come. ▪

4. GO EASY WITH FOOD WHEN COMING OFF ELEMENTAL

Your body will be in a for a big shock when you suddenly start eating again, so take it easy on the food front. Stick to small portions of well-cooked, simple food for the first few days. It might sound boring but, after not eating for a couple of weeks, a few bites of ground beef will sound like a holiday feast.

5. MANAGING SYMPTOMS AND FOOD CRAVINGS

Diffuse peppermint essential oil in the room; it helps with gas and also helps you not go berserk when you smell the food your family is eating in the other room. A hot water bottle on your belly (bonus points for a castor oil pack) helps reduce nausea and belly pains, as does ginger tea. Use visceral manipulation (just massage your abdomen, even if you don't know exactly what you're doing) to help things get moving along.

> "I am currently finding a doctor to order the testing I need to confirm the SIBO. I am following the diet until I do the breath test. I was so glad to find out about the SIBO Solution. I have struggled with IBS for 20 years now. It improved after finding out about my food allergies, but recently reared its ugly head again. Thank you for this valuable information."
>
> — **SHAWN SCHWINDT,** UNITED STATES

¹³ Improving Motility

One of the things I regret most about my first attempt at treating SIBO is not understanding the importance of motility. Dismotility alone could be the cause of your SIBO! Simply speaking, motility means how well things are moving along in the digestive tract. The longer your food sits in the digestive tract, the longer bacteria will be able to feed off of it, causing overgrowth. Motility is not as simple as taking a laxative.

The Migrating Motor Complex

The Migrating Motor Complex is a wave-like series of muscle contractions (a sweeping action) which help move food and waste through the digestive tract. There are actually two different MMC.

The first MMC starts in your stomach and travels through the small intestine.

The second MMC starts duodenum and travels up to the ileocecal valve in the large intestine.

Researchers believe that the MMC acts like a "house-keeping" function. The wave-like movements push undigested food and waste out of our small intestines. When the small intestines are clear of food and waste, then bacteria won't be able to feed off of it. The waves can also clean out excess bacteria too.

During MMC, there are also increases in gastric, biliary, and pancreatic secretions. These secretions probably also help clean out the small intestine of bacteria buildup.[79]

To treat SIBO, you've got to stimulate the MMC and make sure waste is getting out of the small intestine. If you have diarrhea, the idea of stimulating your MMC might seem scary—you don't want more movement happening! But it is important to realize that the MMC doesn't go past the large intestine. It will not worsen your diarrhea.[80]

Though medical researchers have known about the MMC for a long time now, there is a lot we don't know about it and many doctors don't even realize how important it is for gut health and preventing/treating GI diseases like SIBO. Dr. Siebecker says that the MMC is "a key underlying cause which allows SIBO to happen."[80]

It is important to note that the MMC is different than *peristalsis*. Peristalsis is also a wave-like motion through the digestive tract, but it is more like a churning and squeezing action. It occurs after you've eaten food and helps move the food through the GI tract. In the small intestine, peristalsis also sloshes food around so the villi can absorb it. So, we can summarize as peristalsis moves food and MMC makes sure no food waste remains.[81]

Cycles of the MMC

Peristalsis occurs when you *eat food*. By contrast, the MMC only starts when you *haven't eaten food for a while*. Again, this has to do with the apparent role of the MMC as a housekeeper to get out all that undigested food which is why prokinetics before bed are a good idea.

Cycles of the MMC can vary a lot depending on the person. However, research generally shows that the MMC starts about 1½ to 2 hours after not eating. If you are the type of person who "grazes" on food throughout the day, you could be preventing your MMC from starting! Registered Dietician Tamara Duker Freuman says that you should lay off snacking if you've got SIBO or other GI problems related to motility.[82]

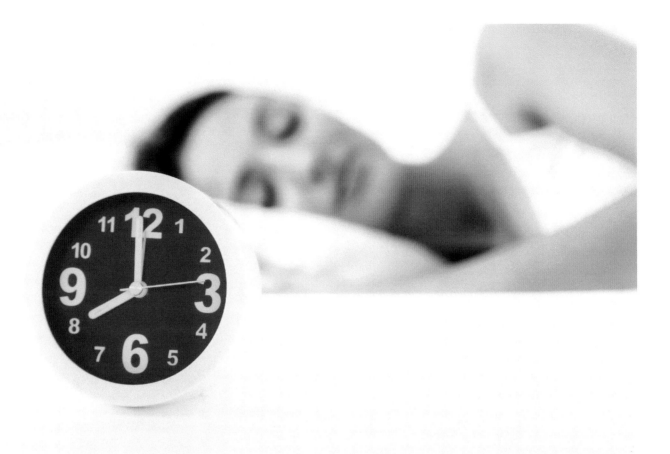

Once it begins, the MMC is divided into 4 phases:

- A calm period lasting about 45 to 60 minutes

- A period of peristaltic contractions which increase in frequency and last for about 30 minutes

- A period of rapid, evenly-spaced peristaltic contractions lasting about 5 to 15 minutes

- A short transition period until phase 1 starts again[79]

One interesting thing to note is that there appears to be a link between MMC cycles and sleep cycles. They appear in similar frequency, have cyclic patterns, and are disrupted by sensory stimuli (such as food with the MMC). There are theories that they are linked, which makes one wonder if lack of sleep could be related to SIBO in this way.[83]

TESTING FOR MMC PROBLEMS

Want to know if your MMC is functioning? There is a test you can take. The test is called IBS Chek and was formulated by Dr. Pimentel, a leading SIBO specialist and author of *A New IBS Solution*. The test is described as a way to diagnose irritable bowel syndrome. However, it is really a test to see whether the MMC is functioning, as an impaired MMC will lead to IBS-like symptoms.

IBS Chek is a quick blood test which looks for the presence of two antibodies: anti-CdtB and anti-vinculin. The presence of these antibodies is a sign that the MMC isn't functioning (because of damage to a protein called vinculin which signals the gut to contract during the MMC). At the time of writing, the test is still very new and is a big breakthrough for diagnosing gut disorders. You can learn more about the test at their website www.ibschek.com.

WAIT AT LEAST 4–5 HOURS BETWEEN MEALS

Do the math: It takes about 1 ½ to 2 hours for the MMC to begin. Then it takes about 1 hour 45 minutes for the MMC to go through all its phases. If you eat during this time, then the MMC will stop. To make sure the MMC is able to do its housekeeping job, you've really got to wait *at least* 3 hours 45 minutes between meals, without grazing or snacking.

Dr. Pimentel, who is a leading expert on SIBO, originally said in his book *A New IBS Solution* that you should wait 3–5 hours between meals. Then he changed his recommendation to 4–5 hours. Everyone's MMC seems to be a bit different. To play it safe, I'd wait for at least 5 hours between meals. That means no snacks, coffee, tea, or anything except water.[80]

CAN'T I JUST TAKE A LAXATIVE?

The problem with laxatives is that they do not trigger the MMC. Some types of laxatives act as stimulants which do trigger peristalsis, so food is moved throughout the GI tract faster—but it won't help clean out any leftover undigested particles which linger about, nor any excess bacteria. Laxatives also don't trigger gastric, biliary, or pancreatic secretions like the MMC does to clean out bacteria.

Other types of laxatives are not stimulants, but rather "stool softeners." They work by drawing water from the intestines and into stool, so your constipation essentially turns to diarrhea. Aside from dehydrating you, these laxatives are made from fiber which could be fermentable—which is a major no-no for SIBO!

Of course, if constipation is a big issue for you, the occasional use of glycerine suppositories is absolutely fine but just know this won't do a thing for your MMC.

USING PROKINETICS TO STIMULATE THE MMC

After you finish SIBO treatment (whether traditional antibiotics, herbal antibiotics or Elemental Diet), you should immediately start taking a prokinetic agent to stimulate the MMC.

I took a prokinetic while doing Elemental Diet and taking herbal antibiotics. Once I finished with Elemental and the herbal antibiotics, I added two more prokinetics. This is the combo which really seemed to do the trick and what ultimately helped me stay clear of SIBO. Check with your doctor to see which combo might be best in your case. These are not the only options.

- **MotilPro:** Take 3 caps before bed and 3 caps 1–2 times a day between meals. (For long term use, 3 before bed may be enough).

- **Iberogast:** Take 20 drops before bed or with meals.

- **Erithromycin—50mg:** This is actually an antibiotic but a really low dose is shown to be highly effective as a prokinetic to stimulate the MMC. You'll need a prescription for it. It comes in 250 mg dose and I cut in 4 so end up with like 67 mg or so which is fine. Take before bed.

Find out where to buy MotilPro and Iberogast on our resource page here www.hollywoodhomestead.com/sibo-solution-resources/

> "I've found The SIBO Solution to be an imperative part of my healing process. I'm almost SIBO free and owe a lot of that to this book."
>
> — **MARISSA CAPUTO,** NEW YORK

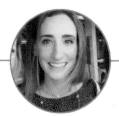

14 Diet Protocols for Treating SIBO

AS WE TALKED ABOUT IN THE PREVIOUS CHAPTERS, ANTIBIOTICS ALONE ARE TERRIBLY INEFFECTIVE AT TREATING SIBO. PATIENTS OFTEN REQUIRE MULTIPLE ROUNDS OF ANTIBIOTICS IN ORDER TO GET THEIR GUT BACTERIAL LEVELS UNDER CONTROL (MY DOCTOR TOLD ME IT PROBABLY WOULD HAVE TAKEN 4 ROUNDS!).

Even after taking multiple courses of antibiotics, SIBO often still comes back. Bacteria can repopulate the small intestine in as little as 2 weeks after completing antibiotics,[84] which is why recurrence rates are around 44% after 9 months.[85] To make sure that SIBO goes away and *stays away*, you've got to address the underlying problems which caused it in the first place. This often means making serious changes to your diet.

IS YOUR DIET CAUSING SIBO?

Remember that bacteria is part of the natural structure of our guts, and it actually serves many important roles in our bodies which range from aiding in digestion to regulating mood. Just like all other living organisms, bacteria have to eat something. And what do bacteria primarily eat? Carbohydrates.

When you eat a low quality diet which is mostly carbohydrates (especially simple carbs like the sugary and starchy foods found in the typical Standard American Diet), bacteria will have a field day. They eat up those excess carbs, proliferate, and then you've got an overgrowth problem on your hand. It certainly doesn't help that the SAD diet also is full of inflammatory foods like gluten and seed oils which can damage the lining of the stomach and decrease stomach acid production. As we talked about in chapter 03 about the Causes of SIBO, stomach acid is important for regulating and killing bacteria in the gut. Without enough stomach acid, you will also have undigested particles of food in your small intestine, which the bacteria can then eat.

DIETARY PROTOCOLS FOR TREATING SIBO

There are 4 main dietary approaches to treating SIBO. They vary significantly, but are all based on one common principle: *starve the bacteria and/or don't re-feed it.*

LOW FODMAP DIET FOR SIBO

FODMAP stands for Fermentable Oligosaccharides, Disaccharides, Monosaccharides, and Polyols, which are the four classes of fermentable sugars/sugar alcohols. The Low FODMAP diet was originally derived as a dietary treatment for IBS but can be adapted for treating SIBO.

The idea behind the Low FODMAP diet is that you get rid of foods which contribute to intestinal fermentation. Low FODMAP diet is very effective in treating gastrointestinal conditions like IBD and IBS. However, it is important to note that the Low FODMAP diet *does not* restrict polysaccharide and disaccharide sources of carbs such as grains, starch, starchy vegetables, and sucrose. These carbs are normally well-absorbed, but with SIBO they aren't absorbed well and bacteria can feed off of them and worsen the problem. So, to treat SIBO, these carbs must also be removed.[86, 87]

Note: It's **LOW** FODMAP, not **NO** FODMAP, so try not to drive yourself too insane.

SCD Diet for SIBO

SCD stands for Specific Carbohydrate Diet. It was originally developed by a pediatrician for treating Celiac Disease and was later popularized by Elaine Gottschall in her book *Breaking the Vicious Cycle*, which you can find listed on our resource page here www.hollywoodhomestead.com/sibo-solution-resources/. SCD limits complex carbs (disaccharides and polysaccharides), lactose, sucrose and other man-made (read: crappy) ingredients. These ingredients are harmful to the digestive system and lead to yeast overgrowth, bacteria overgrowth, and inflammation. According to data from surveys, SCD has a 75% to 84% success rate.[88]

Here are some examples of SCD foods:

ALLOWED:

- Meat

- Kale, lettuce, peas, peppers, mushrooms

- Ghee

- Some legumes

- Most spices

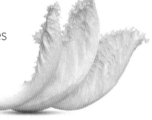

NOT ALLOWED:

- Cereal grains (wheat, corn, oats, rye, etc.)

- Processed meat

- Canned fruits and vegetables

- Soy, chickpeas, fava beans, bean sprouts

- Commercial milk and dairy products

- Potatoes, yams, sweet potatoes

GAPS Diet for SIBO

GAPS stands for Gut and Psychology Syndrome. The diet was created by Dr. Natasha Campbell-McBride. It is based on the idea that all disease starts in the gut—which is supported by the fact that 90% of all cells and genetic material in the human body belongs to gut flora. Campbell-McBride says that modern life damages the gut flora and leads to diseases including autism, ADD, epilepsy, depression, as well as many other diseases.

GAPS diet is similar to SCD diet, but allows/excludes a few different items and also has a very clear outline. There are seven phases to the GAPS diet. The introductory stage is basically a fast which allows very little food, room temperature water, and probiotics. As you move through the phases, you are allowed to add more foods to the diet—such as egg yolks, avocado, and squash. There are some foods which are not allowed at any phase of the diet. GAPS diet also heavily focuses on detoxing.[89]

NOT ALLOWED DURING ANY PHASE:

- Sugars (other than fruit)

- Potatoes, rice, flour

- Wheat

- Dairy

While many have experienced great results such as reversing food allergies and improving symptoms of behavioral and mood disorders with GAPS, there isn't any scientific evidence supporting GAPS diet for SIBO. Because the diet removes starches and certain sugars, as well as difficult-to-digest foods like beans, it can help reduce inflammation and intestinal fermentation. However, the diet does not remove high FODMAP foods. These foods act much like sugars and starches, meaning that you could still be feeding the bacteria in the gut. For this reason, even GAPS diet will have to be adapted if it is going to be used to effectively treat SIBO.[90]

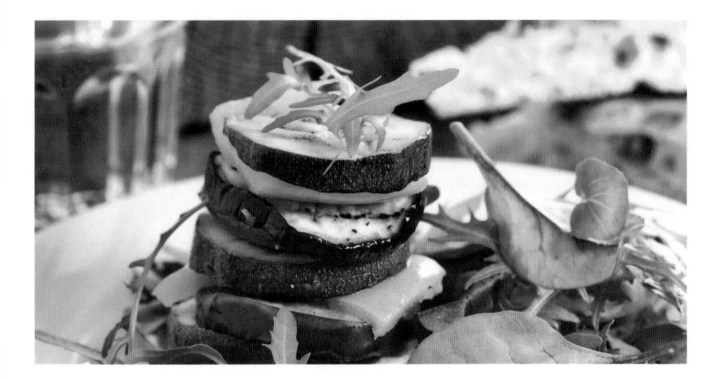

CEDARS-SINAI DIET FOR PREVENTING SIBO

The other diets mentioned above are used for *treating* SIBO. By contrast, the Cedar-Sinai Diet is designed to *prevent* SIBO. It was devised Dr. Mark Pimentel, Director of the Gastrointestinal Motility Program at Cedars-Sinai Medical Center. The diet isn't as strict as the ones listed above, but follows the same general principles: you've got to reduce foods which are hard for your body to digest so bacteria don't end up using them as food. Pimentel's diet also advises against frequent eating because this can affect the migrating motor complex which helps empty and clean the bowels.[91] He outlines the details in his book *A New IBS Solution,* which you can find on our resource page here www.hollywoodhomestead.com/sibo-solution-resources/.

> "I am currently free of SIBO after following your advice last May. Thank you!"
>
> — **CAROL**, NOVA SCOTIA, CANADA

Key Points of the Cedars-Sinai Diet:

- Avoid sweeteners like corn syrup, mannitol, sorbitol, lactose, and sucralose

- Avoid dairy

- Limit beans, lentils and peas

- Drink 8 cups of water per day

- Eat protein like beef, fish, poultry, and eggs in body-appropriate portion sizes

- Some carbohydrates are okay, but must experiment with how your body reacts to them

- Eat fruits in moderation

- Eat non-starchy vegetables

- Coffee and tea are okay in moderation; soda should be avoided

The protocol also involves taking a prokinetic drug to improve motility and supplementing with hydrochloric acid, if deficient.

15 The SIBO Diet

WHEN TREATING AND PREVENTING SIBO WITH DIET, THE MOST IMPORTANT THING TO REMEMBER IS TO AVOID ANY FOOD WHICH BACTERIA LOVE TO EAT. THIS BASICALLY MEANS AVOIDING MOST CARBOHYDRATES, WHICH ARE REFERRED TO AS "FERMENTABLES." THE ONLY CARBS WHICH BACTERIA DON'T REALLY EAT ARE INSOLUBLE FIBER.

A combination of the Low FODMAPs diet and SCD Diet is considered best for treating SIBO. On their own, each of these diets has its flaws. For example, SCD (which was originally created for treating Celiac) allows garlic—which is highly fermentable. Low FOD-MAP (which is primarily used for treating IBS) allows ingredients like dairy, soy, and grains—which will also wreak havoc on your gut. By combining SCD and Low FODMAP, you get rid of most of the fermentables. The combo is called "The SIBO-Specific Diet".

However, even SIBO Specific isn't exactly ideal because it allows a some things which aren't great for your health—such as the artificial sweeteners aspartame and saccharine. These are things I wouldn't recommend for anyone to eat, with or without SIBO. The diet also allows legumes which are not ideal for someone trying to heal their gut lining.

When you have SIBO, your gut is under severe inflammation and might even already have holes in it (leaky gut). You want to make sure you aren't consuming anything which is going to irritate your gut. Even better, you want to consume food which is going to *heal* your gut.

For these reasons, the best diet for treating sibo is a combination of:

Low FODMAP + SCD + Paleo/Primal

The Low FODMAP and SCD diets take care of the fermentable and pro-inflammatory foods which will feed bacteria. The Paleo diet will take care of all those unnatural foods which wreak havoc on your gut health (not to mention the rest of your health).

THE SIBO DIET PROTOCOL

The moment you confirm you've got SIBO, you will want to put yourself on The SIBO Diet. Even if you are taking antibiotics for SIBO, you will still want to attack it with a dietary approach. Again, the goal isn't just to get rid of bacteria, but to *keep it away* and *heal your gut.*

HOW LONG DO YOU NEED TO BE ON THE SIBO DIET?

Follow The SIBO Diet all during treatment (unless you are doing Elemental during which you won't be eating anything). Yes, I know it is hard to make major dietary changes to your life, but your health is SO worth it. And after you get over the initial transition period, you will probably never want to go back to eating the foods that give you symptoms, or at the very least proceed with caution.

After you cure SIBO, I'd recommend sticking to The SIBO Diet for about 3 months. You can gradually try small amounts of fermentable foods but certain foods that have no nutritional value I'd advise staying away from for the long haul (we really don't need junk like corn syrup and hydrogenated oil when we can just use more nutrient dense foods like honey and olive oil). When adding a fermentable food back to your diet, try to make it one that is nourishing and/or a food that you miss and really makes you happy. Your mental health is just as important as your physical health, and you don't want to feel like you are depriving yourself.

Over time, you will customize *your best diet*. This "best" diet will likely evolve over the upcoming months or even years. You'll find out which foods are worth eating for you, and which foods you are happy to give up.

For example, I've noticed that milk (lactose) does not agree with me right now. I had to suffer through several cappuccinos at my favorite café before I was ready to accept this hard truth. It isn't likely a life sentence but, for now, I'm laying off the cappuccinos to avoid those tummy troubles. On the other hand, I've learned that I can order a glass of wine without experiencing any symptoms so that's a treat that I'm happy to be able to have on occasion. Find what flexibility works best for you. Chances are no two SIBO diets will look alike.

How Strict Do You Need to Be on The SIBO Diet?

During treatment, I would try to follow The SIBO Diet as closely as you can. Antibiotics (both pharmaceutical and herbal) have a really low success rate for treating SIBO, and you don't want to decrease your chances of success by eating foods which will feed the bacteria in your gut. This might require more time than you are used to in the kitchen and shopping and prepping for foods. For helpful advice on how to upgrade your diet and make it work for your lifestyle when you are busy with kids, travel, work, etc, read *Paleo Made Easy*. You can find it on the resource page here: www.hollywoodhomestead.com/sibo-solution-resources/.

After your breath tests finally come back as negative for SIBO, you will still want to stick to The SIBO Diet for 3 months. This will allow your gut to heal and your bacteria levels to normalize.

Ideally, you would stick to The SIBO Diet perfectly for the 3 months following treatment. But here's the thing:

as mentioned before, stress is the leading cause of SIBO and a huge cause of recurrence. Stress is probably what got you here in the first place, so stressing about food isn't going to help you fight SIBO!

Further, The SIBO Diet isn't like other elimination diets (such as the Paleo Autoimmune Protocol) where you really need to follow the diet 100% in order to make it effective. It is not necessary to avoid *all* FODMAPs—the poison is really in the *amount*. A scoop of avocado might be fine, but an entire avocado might destroy you.

Honestly, my diet was not perfect after finishing the second round of Elemental and the concurrent course of herbal antibiotics, which is why I was shocked when my test results came back negative.

The most important thing to remember is to not drive yourself crazy trying to follow The SIBO Diet 100% accurately, 100% of the time. Just do the best you can. Avoiding something as common as garlic when eating out is almost impossible. But, as much as I enjoy it, garlic was my kryptonite and something I haven't been brave enough to try reintroducing yet.

The only time I'd say you should be super strict is if you've got a confirmed autoimmune disease and really need to watch your diet. Otherwise, I'd say do your best to stick to the foods in the chart and slowly introduce other foods when you are ready.

What Do You Eat on The SIBO Diet?

The following table shows you foods which are okay to eat on The SIBO Diet and ones which are fermentable and should be avoided or eaten with caution. Remember, with SIBO, it isn't the food itself which is the problem but rather the dosage. You don't have to drive yourself crazy avoiding all of the foods on the "no" list—just consume them in moderation and see how your body reacts.

Not sure what to cook on The SIBO Diet? In the recipes section on page 77, you can find all sorts of easy meal ideas which won't feed the bacteria in your gut and can even help gut healing.

SIBO Food Lists

MEATS

YES (NOTE AMOUNTS)	NO
Bacon with honey	Bacon with sugar or HFCS
Broth—homemade meat or marrow bones (no cartilage)	Broth: homemade bone/cartilage
Beef	Deli/processed meat with sugar, carrageenan, high FODMAP or SCD illegal additives
Eggs	
Fish	
Game	
Lamb	
Organ meats	
Pork	
Poultry	
Seafood	

FATS & OILS

YES (NOTE AMOUNTS)	NO
Bacon fat	Soybean oil
Butter	Seed oils: canola, walnut, grapeseed, sesame seed, safflower, sunflower, corn
Coconut oil	Vegetable shortening
Cod liver oil & Fish oil	Margarine
Duck fat	
Garlic-infused oil	
Ghee	
Lard & Tallow	
Medium chain triglyceride/MCT oil	
Macadamia oil	
Olive oil	
Palm oil	

Download an updated list to keep handy or print out for FREE here:
www.hollywoodhomestead.com/sibo-detox/

YES (NOTE AMOUNTS)	NO
Artichoke hearts ⅛ c	Artichoke hearts > ⅛ c
Arugula	Asparagus
Bamboo shoots	Avocado
Beet 2 slices	Bean sprouts
Bok Choy 1 c /85g	Beet > 2 slices
Broccoli ½ c/1.6oz	Bok Choy > 1c
Brussels Sprouts 2 ea	Broccoli > ½ c
Cabbage 1 c/98g	Brussels Sprouts > 2 ea
Cabbage: Savoy ½ c	Butternut Squash
Carrot	Cabbage: Savoy ¾ c
Celery root/Celeriac	Canned vegetables
Chives	Cauliflower
Cucumber	Celery
Eggplant	Corn
Endive	Fennel bulb > ½ c, leaves 1 c
Fennel bulb ½ c, leaves 1 c	Garlic
Green beans 10 ea/2.5oz	Jerusalem artichoke
Greens: lettuce, collard, chard, kale, spinach	Mushrooms
Leek ½ stalk	Okra
Olives	Onions
Parsnip	Peas, green > ¼ c
Peas, green ¼ c	Pepper: chili 40g
Peppers: bell/sweet	Potato: sweet
Peppers: chili 11cm/28g	Potato: white/all colors
Radicchio 12 leaves	Scallions: white part
Radish	Seaweeds
Rutabaga	Shallot
Scallion: green part	Snow peas > 5 pods
Snow peas 5 pods	Spinach > 15 leaves/150g
Squash Kabocha, Sunburst, Yellow, Zucchini ¾ c	Starch powder: all (arrowroot, corn, potato, rice, tapioca)
Squash: butternut ¼ c	Sugar Snap Peas
Tomato	Taro
	Tomato: soup/juice, sundried
	Turnip
	Water Chestnut
	Yam
	Yellow Zucchini > ¾ c
	Yucca

Download an updated list to keep handy
or print out for FREE here:
www.hollywoodhomestead.com/sibo-detox/

FRUITS

YES (NOTE AMOUNTS)	NO
Banana—fresh, dried	Apple
Berries: blueberry < 80 ea, boysenberry, strawberry, raspberry 10 ea/19g	Apricot
Carambola	Avocado
Citrus: lemon, lime, oranges, tangelos, tangerine	Berries: cranberry, blueberry > 80/100g, blackberry, raspberry > 10ea
Current, dried 1Tbsp	Citrus: grapefruit
Dragon fruit	Current, dried > 1 Tbsp
Durian	Custard Apple
Grapes	Date, dried
Guava	Fig, dried
Kiwifruit	Longon > 5ea
Longon 5 ea/15g	Lychee
Melon: cantaloupe/rock, honeydew ½ c/100g	Mango
Papaya/Paw Paw	Melon: honeydew > ½c
Passion fruit 4 pulps/100g	Nectarine
Pineapple	Papaya, dried
Pomegranate ½ ea/38g, ¼ c seeds	Passion fruit > 4 pulps
Prickly Pear	Pineapple, dried
Rambutan 2 ea/31g	Peach
Rhubarb	Pear
Jam/Jelly—homemade from allowable fruits—see fruit list (no pectin, sugar)	Pear: nashi
Tomato	Persimmon
	Plum
	Pomegranat > ½ ea, > ¼ c seeds
	Prunes
	Plantain
	Raisins
	Rambutan > 2 ea
	Tamarillo
	Watermelon
	Canned fruit in High FODMAP fruit juice
	Jam/Jelly—commercial

Download an updated list to keep handy or print out for FREE here:
www.hollywoodhomestead.com/sibo-detox/

Nuts & Seeds

Yes (note amounts)	No
Almonds 10 ea/0.42oz, flour 2 Tbsp	Almonds > 10 ea, > 2 Tbsp flour
Coconut: flour/shredded ¼ c, milk (w/no thickeners)	Chestnuts
Hazelnuts 10 ea/15g	Cashews
Macadamia 20 ea/40g	Coconut milk with thickeners (guar gum, carageenan)
Pecans 10 ea/22g	Chia seeds
Pine nuts 1 Tbsp/14g	Flaxseeds
Pumpkin seeds 2 Tbsp/23g	Hazelnuts > 10 ea
Sesame seeds 1 Tbsp/11g	Macadamia > 20 ea
Sunflower seeds 2 tsp/6g	Pecans > 10 ea
Walnuts 10 ea/30g	Pine nuts > 1 Tbsp
	Pistachios
	Pumpkin seeds > 2 Tbsp
	Sesame seeds > 1Tbsp
	Seed flour
	Sunflower seeds > 2 Tbsp
	Walnuts > 10 ea

Dairy

Yes (note amounts)	No
Butter	Cream—lactasetreated
Cheese: aged 1mo+, dry curd cottage cheese, yogurt cheese/labneh	Cheese: cream cheese, cottage cheese, fresh cheese (feta, cheve, fresh mozzarella), ricotta
Ghee	Kefir—commercial, homemade 24 hour
Sour cream—homemade 24 hour	Cream
Yogurt—homemade 24 hour	Milk
	Sour cream—commercial
	Yogurt—commercial

Download an updated list to keep handy or print out for FREE here:
www.hollywoodhomestead.com/sibo-detox/

BEVERAGES AND ALCOHOL

YES (NOTE AMOUNTS)	NO
COMMON DRINKS	**COMMON DRINKS**
Coffee 1 c/day (weak)	Coffee > 1 c/day (weak)
Cranberry juice-pure	Fruit juice from Low FODMAP fruits > ⅓ c/100ml
Orange juice, fresh ½ c/125ml	Fruit juice from High FODMAP fruits
Fruit juice from Low FODMAP fruits ⅓ c/100ml	Coffee substitutes
Tea: black (weak), camomile, ginger, green, hibiscus, lemongrass, mate, mint, oolong (weak), rooibos/rooibos chai, rose hip	Soda (fructose, sucrose)
Water	Tea: chicory root, licorice, pau d'arco
	Tea: green > 2 c/day
	Seltzer/Carbonated beverages (CO_2/gas)
ALCOHOL	**ALCOHOL**
Occasionally in moderate amounts: Bourbon, Gin, Vodka, Whiskey/Scotch, Wine	Rum: light/gold, dark
	Brandy
	Hard Cider
	Liqueurs/Cordials
	Sherry
	Tequila
	Wine: dessert/sweet, sake, sparkling, port

Download an updated list to keep handy or print out for FREE here:
www.hollywoodhomestead.com/sibo-detox/

Condiments and Seasonings

YES (NOTE AMOUNTS)	NO
All spices (except onion & garlic)	Asafoetida powder
Garlic-infused oil	Chicory root (leaves ok)
Ginger (fresh & dried)	Cocoa/chocolate unsweetened
Mayonnaise, homemade or commercial w/honey	Gums/Carrageenan/Thickeners
Mustard—without garlic	Sauces or Marinades with High FODMAP/SCD illegal items
Pickles/Relish—no sweetener or garlic	Soy Sauce/Tamari
Tabasco (McIlhennyCo)	Spices: onion & garlic powder
Wasabi—pure	Venegar: balsamic
Vinegar: apple cider, distilled/white, red & white wine	Baking powder

Sweeteners

YES (NOTE AMOUNTS)	NO
Glucose/Dextrose	Agave syrup
Honey: alfalfa, cotton, clover, raspberry 2 Tbsp	Barley Malt syrup
Stevia—pure (no inulin) in small amounts, occasionally	Cane sugar (Rapadura, Sucanat)
	Coconut sugar
	Fructose, powdered
	Honey: blackberry, buckwheat, citrus/orange blossom, acacia, sage, tupelo
	Honey: raspberry > 2 Tbsp
	High-fructose corn syrup
	Maple syrup
	Molasses
	Sugar/Sucrose
	Sucralose
	Polyols/Sugar alcohol: isomalt, erythritol, lactitol, maltitol, mannitol, sorbitol, xylitol

Download an updated list to keep handy or print out for FREE here:
www.hollywoodhomestead.com/sibo-detox/

¹⁶ Preventing Recurrence

IF YOU ARE READING THIS BOOK, I WOULDN'T BE SURPRISED IF YOU HAVE ALREADY UNDERGONE MULTIPLE BOUTS OF ANTIBIOTICS, WITH DOSAGES OR REGIMENS CHANGING EACH TIME. SYMPTOMS MIGHT CLEAR UP TEMPORARILY, ONLY TO RETURN IN A FEW WEEKS OR MONTHS. SIBO HAS AN INCREDIBLY HIGH RECURRENCE RATE, AND IT IS VERY IMPORTANT THAT YOU UNDERSTAND THIS BEFORE YOU SET ABOUT TREATING THE DISEASE.

SIBO RECURRENCE RATES

Treating SIBO isn't about getting rid of all the bacteria in your small intestine (you need bacteria there!). It is about getting your gut bacteria at a healthy balance. You will always have bacteria in your gut, and bacteria is a living thing. It will reproduce. If the conditions of your gut are healthy after finishing a bout of antibiotics, then the bacteria will stay at healthy levels. If not, then **bacteria can begin to repopulate again in as little as two weeks.**[92] Since antibiotics don't address the underlying problems which caused the bacteria to get out of control in the first place, recurrence is almost inevitable.

According to one study[85] in which patients were treated with rifaximin, patients experienced these rates of recurrence:

- 12.6% after 3 months

- 27.5% after 6 months

- 43.7% after 9 months

Keep in mind that a single round of antibiotics is only effective in about half of cases, so your chances of beating SIBO with just one round of antibiotics is really low.[1]

WHY IS THIS SO IMPORTANT?

Because it very important to realize that you've got to treat the underlying causes of SIBO, not just the bacterial overgrowth!

Taking antibiotics every single time your SIBO comes back is NOT the solution! Aside from being a major annoyance which includes unpleasant symptoms, frequent doctors' visits and continual testing, the bacteria in your gut could become resistant to the SIBO antibiotics. When this happens, you are going to have to take even higher dosages of antibiotics and/or different types of antibiotics.[69]

Who wants to be a guinea pig for every pharmaceutical in the book? I know I don't.

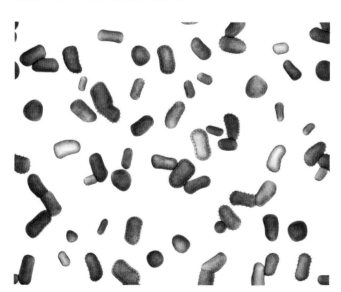

Steps to Prevent SIBO Recurrence

1. Reduce Stress

The most important thing you can do to prevent SIBO recurrence is *reduce stress*. Stress isn't just the #1 cause of SIBO, it is also a leading cause of conditions which contribute to SIBO—like how stress causes gut inflammation, which can set the stage for bacterial overgrowth. I suggest you re-read through the Causes of SIBO chapter of this book on page 18 to see how everything comes back to stress.

2. Eat a Real Foods Diet

Along with reducing stress, you will need to maintain a healthy diet. You don't have to stick to the SIBO diet forever, but you will want to adhere to its core principles: *avoid excess carbs and avoid foods which harm the gut.*

The worst thing you can do for your gut (and body and mind) is to eat the Standard American Diet (appropriately called SAD). This diet is high in foods which irritate the lining of the gut, reduce stomach acid (which you need to keep bacteria levels in check), and are low in nutrients.

Diet is too big of an issue to discuss in detail here. For starters, I'd recommend getting rid of ALL processed foods and gluten. My family and I follow a paleo diet and I credit it directly to solving numerous health problems we've had, including weight problems, acne and eczema, low immunity, and digestion problems. If you are interested in upgrading your diet, read *Paleo Made Easy*. The book has useful information on which foods to eat and avoid, shopping advice, cooking tips, and more. You can find the book listed on our resource page here: www.hollywoodhomestead.com/sibo-solution-resources/

3. Take Probiotics

As Nutritionist Angela Pifer points out, SIBO treatment usually doesn't include probiotics. The rationale for this is that probiotics are bacteria, so you don't want to add more bacteria to your gut when you have SIBO.

Pifer advocates taking probiotics because, in most cases of SIBO, probiotics are not the type of bacteria causing problems. They are the "good bacteria" which help reduce inflammation, maintain proper gut pH, and even help kill off the "bad guys" which shouldn't be there. Further, she notes that if you are taking antibiotics for SIBO, then you are going to kill off the good bacteria in your gut along with the bad. You will need to replenish this, or else your gut flora will remain unbalanced and SIBO is bound to recur.

Bear in mind that there haven't been much research on probiotics for treating and preventing SIBO, but the few studies which are out there are promising.[93] You can add probiotic supplements to your daily regimen. We list some on the resource page here: www.hollywoodhomestead.com/sibo-solution-resources/

But make sure your probiotics don't include PREbiotics!

If you just grab any probiotics off the shelf in hopes they will help keep SIBO at bay, you might be surprised to find your symptoms get worse. The reason for this is because many probiotics contain *prebiotics*. Prebiotics are the fiber which probiotics eat. But the bad bacteria also happen to love prebiotics! The bacteria eat this fiber and overgrowth can occur/recur. So, if you are going to take probiotics for SIBO, you must make sure they do not include any prebiotics, fillers, or other junk.[94]

4. Increase Stomach Acid

If you remember from the Causes of SIBO chapter, one of the leading causes of SIBO is not having enough stomach acid. That's right—we *want* stomach acid! Stomach acid is responsible for breaking down food. No, too much stomach acid does *not* cause heartburn or acid reflux. It is *too little* stomach acid which causes heartburn and acid reflux.

If you don't have enough stomach acid, then you will have a lot of undigested food particles in your small intestine. Bacteria will feed off of these food particles and overgrowth will occur. That means inflammation, gas, and a lot of pressure on your gut. All that pressure causes your stomach acid to push up into your esophagus, i.e. *heartburn*.

How do you know if you have low stomach acid (hypochlorhydria)?

According to certified nutritionist Dr. Joseph Debe the Heidelberg Stomach Acid test is the best, most reliable way of testing for low stomach acid. Unfortunately, the test costs about $350 to perform. If you don't want to spring for this test, then you can try these two cheaper options.

- **The Baking Soda Test:** Mix ¼ tsp of baking soda in 4–6oz of cold water. Drink it first thing in the morning before eating or drinking anything. Time how long it takes you to belch. Stop after 5 minutes. If you have enough stomach acid, you should belch within 2 or 3 minutes. This isn't very accurate, but it is cheap and easy.

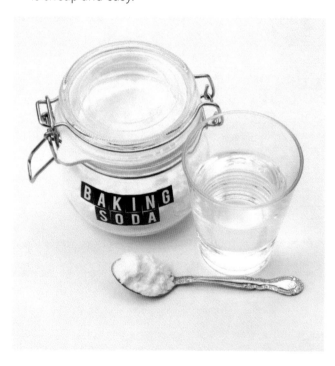

- **The Betaine HCL Challenge Test:** Buy some Betaine HCL tablets with pepsin. Eat at least 6oz of meat. In the middle of the meal, take 1 of the Betaine HCL tablets. Finish the meal and pay attention to your body throughout the rest of the day. If you don't notice any changes, then you probably have low stomach acid levels. If you notice stomach distress, then your stomach acid levels are probably fine.

While you are at it, you are going to want to stop using all those antacids so your stomach acid levels can get back to normal and bacteria can stabilize.

5. STIMULATE THE MIGRATING MOTOR COMPLEX

As we talked about in chapter 13, the Migrating Motor Complex is the wave-like motions that sweep through the intestines and help clean the gut of excess bacteria and undigested food particles. One of the leading causes of SIBO is an improperly working MMC. When your MMC isn't doing its job, then food is going to sit inside your small intestine too long (constipation!) and bacteria will have a field day on it.

There are a few ways to stimulate the MMC. The most important one is to avoid stress, as stress will shut off the MMC. You will also want to follow these tips:

- Don't eat snacks between meals (to allow plenty of time for your intestines to flush out food)

- Get plenty of sleep

- Try acupuncture for MMC

- Take prokinetic drugs (such as those recommended on the resource page here: www.hollywoodhomestead.com/sibo-solution-resources/)

6. HEAL THE INTESTINAL LINING

SIBO can do a lot of damage to your intestinal lining, which in turn can cause severe problems like leaky gut. So, to cure SIBO for good, you will also need to repair your intestinal lining. This is a hefty subject which we will get into the next chapter but half, if not more, of the work of repairing the gut is done by simply eliminating the offender, which in this case is the overgrowth!

> "It's been 5 ½ weeks since I started the SIBO diet and the first time in years I feel good!"
>
> **— DAWN**

¹⁷ Healing the Gut

WHEN YOU HAVE SIBO, THE BACTERIAL OVERGROWTH CREATES AN INFLAMMATORY RESPONSE IN THE INTESTINAL MUCOSA. THE INFLAMMATION NOT ONLY MAKES SYMPTOMS WORSE, BUT CAN LEAD TO LEAKY GUT SYNDROME.²⁹ TO CURE SIBO, YOU NEED TO MAKE SURE THAT YOU ARE ALSO TAKING STEPS TO HEAL YOUR GUT FROM THE DAMAGE WHICH HAS BEEN DONE.

WHAT IS LEAKY GUT SYNDROME?

When you eat food, your digestive system breaks the food down into tiny parts. These digested particles pass through the lining of the stomach and into our bloodstream. The gut is designed in a way so only fully broken down food particles can pass through. Think of it like a window screen. The screen lets air through but stops bugs from getting inside. Our gut linings are like this screen, allowing nutrients through but stopping undigested food particles from getting past.

If the lining of the gut gets damaged, then holes can form. Particles of undigested food are able to escape through those holes (hence the name leaky gut) and into our bloodstream.

Anything which causes inflammation can lead to leaky gut. This includes chronic stress, certain medications, antibiotics, GMOs, birth control pills, and excessive alcohol consumption. The big culprit of leaky gut though is usually *food sensitivities*.⁹⁵

If you only exposed yourself to these pro-inflammatory conditions occasionally, your gut might be able to heal itself, but many of us lead lifestyles in which our guts are *constantly* subjected to inflammation. Just think how many people eat cereal for breakfast, a sandwich for lunch, and then top off all that gluten with some spaghetti for dinner! Now think how many people are constantly stressed out by work and rushing around. Then factor in all the chemical additives in "foodstuff", prescription medications, GMOs ...

Obviously, having holes in your gut is *no bueno*. But it is worse than you might realize. When bits of undigested food escape through the gut, they get into the bloodstream. Our immune systems then attack these food particles. The problem is that some of these food particles resemble substances in our bodies, so the immune system gets confused *and starts attacking itself.* That means autoimmune diseases. **Yes, all autoimmune disease starts with leaky gut syndrome—and SIBO leads to leaky gut!**

And things get even worse from here.

When your gut is damaged, your stomach membranes don't produce gastric acid efficiently.⁹⁶ Without enough acid, you can develop bacterial overgrowth (or, if you already have it, the overgrowth gets worse). Bacterial overgrowth can then make leaky gut worse. In this sense, SIBO and Leaky Gut aren't just an "A leads to B" thing; they are part of a vicious cycle.

Inflammation	→	Leaky gut	→	Reduced Stomach Acid	→	Excess Bacteria Causes More Inflammation	→	Worsened Leaky Gut

No matter what you do to get SIBO bacteria levels in check, you aren't going to fully overcome from those digestive problems if you've got a damaged gut lining. Healing your gut is a big topic, and I discuss it a lot more deeply in my eBook *The Gelatin Secret* (which you can find on the resource page here: www.hollywoodhome-stead.com/sibo-solution-resources/) but here are the basic steps you need to take to heal your intestinal lining.

1. ELIMINATE PRO-INFLAMMATORY FOODS

A food sensitivity is any food which irritates your gut and leads to inflammation. Food allergies also cause irritation and inflammation. However, the difference between the two is that, with an allergy, your body mistakenly thinks something is a harmful invader. The body releases its soldiers (histamines) to fight the invader, causing symptoms.

Food sensitivities don't cause the immediate reaction as allergies. This makes them harder to pinpoint. One day, for example, you might be fine eating corn. But, as you continue to eat corn, all the irritation adds up to the point where you experience symptoms and yet you still might not know what food is causing it because it crept up on you over time. The best way to pinpoint food sensitivities is to do an elimination diet for 30 days. To do this, you remove suspected food sensitivities (the most common ones are gluten, corn, eggs, and dairy). After 30 days, you introduce them one at a time to see if you experience a reaction. In her book *The Paleo Approach,* Dr. Sarah Ballantyne talks in depth about how to do an elimination diet. The book is mostly in reference to autoimmune diseases, but I recommend it to anyone with health issues as a must-have encyclopedia of sorts. You can find the book on our resource page here www.hollywoodhomestead.com/sibo-solution-resources/

Many of us on the Standard American Diet eat nothing but gut irritants all day. There are a LOT of gut irritants, but the big ones are:[53]

- Gluten

- Grains (including, but not limited to those containing gluten)

- Nuts

- Legumes

- Eggs

- Caffeine

- Alcohol

- Nightshades

- Processed sugar

- Processed foods

- GMOs (genetically modified organisms)

The first step in repairing your gut lining and solving SIBO for good is to ELIMINATE ALL PROCESSED FOOD. It shouldn't even be considered food but rather *food stuff.* So no more TV dinners, boxes of cookies, or grocery store items with ingredients you can't even pronounce. Your gut doesn't need these items. Your body certainly doesn't need them either!

2. DECREASE OMEGA-6 TO OMEGA-3 RATIO

You've probably heard about Omega-3 and all of its health benefits. What a lot of those health articles gloss over is the fact that it isn't enough to just increase Omega-3. You've got to simultaneously decrease the amount of Omega-6 in your diet.

This is a huge topic that requires a discussion about how the body converts Omega-3 into the fatty acids EPA and DHA, and how Omega-3 and Omega-6 compete for the same pathways. Here are some key points that you need to know about Omega-3 : Omega-6 ratios.

- Anthropological research shows that our hunter-gatherer ancestors ate Omega-3 and Omega-6 in a 1:1 ratio

- Today, people eat Omega-3 and Omega-6 in ratios of about 1:10 to 1:20!

- A diet high in Omega-3 and low in Omega-6 will *reduce inflammation*

A diet low in Omega-3 and high in Omega-6 will *increase inflammation*

Ideally aim for a 1:4 Omega-3 to Omega-6 ratio (1:1 would be better, but that is probably not achievable unless you are Eskimo and eating wild salmon all day!)

People following a typical American diet are getting about 20% of their calories from a single source: *soybean oil.* Guess what soybean oil is high in? Yep, Omega-6. The same is true of other common oils, such as sunflower oil or corn oil. To make things worse, these oils oxidize quickly, which can turn them into harmful trans fats! Heart disease anyone?[97, 98]

One of the best things you can do for your gut and overall health is to cut out all those pro-inflammatory cooking oils. What should you cook with instead? My personal favorite is tallow, which has an Omega-3:6 ratio of about 1:6, which is a huge improvement over sunflower oil which has a ratio of about 1:200 or safflower oil which has no Omega-3 at all.Ghee (clarified butter) is also a great alternative to cooking oil.[99, 100, 101, 102]

Another important thing you can do to reduce Omega-6 is switch to grass-fed beef and wild-caught salmon. Cows eating their natural diet of grass instead of corn have much higher levels of Omega-3. How much higher? Grain-fed beef can have Omega-6:3 ratios exceeding 20:1 whereas grass-fed beef is around 3:1. With salmon, farmed salmon may contain just half of the omega 3s as wild-caught salmon. I get that most people probably aren't going to eat wild salmon all day long to optimize their Omega-3:6 ratios. It may be worth considering a supplement, such as Thorne brand's Super EPA.[103, 104] You can find it listed on the resource page here: www.hollywoodhomestead.com/sibo-solution-resources/

1. NOURISH THE GUT LINING

Getting rid of gut irritants and optimizing Omega-3 to Omega-6 ratios is a start. If you want to speed up gut healing though, you've got to provide your gut with nutrients it needs to heal. One of the absolute best superfoods you can consume for gut healing is *bone broth*.

Real bone broth is made from boiled down bones and connective tissues. **With SIBO, it is important that you only make bone broth with marrow and meat bones.** Cartilage bones (such as knuckle bones) rate high on FODMAP and need to be avoided. You can find a recipe for SIBO-friendly bone broth on page 78.[105]

Once you've boiled down the bones, you are left with a liquid which is very rich in nutrients. Most importantly, bone broth is also rich in gelatin. It turns out that gelatin acts like spackle to fill the holes in your gut. No wonder bone broth has long been considered the go-to remedy for digestive ailments! Steven Horne (AHG and IIPA) and Thomas Easton (AHG) recommend drinking about 1–4 cups of bone broth daily to repair your gut from SIBO. You'll probably want to start slowly though and gradually increase your dosage, letting your body guide you and starting with marrow bone broth before you gradually introduce gelatinous broth made from cartilage.[106]

If you really hate the taste of bone broth, you can consume real gelatin instead (I'm not talking about the Jell-o packets you buy at the supermarket which are made from byproducts and chemical additives—avoid those like the plague!) Real gelatin is FODMAPs safe. Some people still find it difficult to digest so take it slow and increase the dose as your body allows.[107]

There are only a couple of brands of real gelatin that I know of. You can use it to make tasty treats like gummies, smoothies, and much more. You can find loads of easy gelatin recipes in my book *The Gelatin Secret.*[108] You can find the the the book and my favorite brands of gelatin listed on the resource page here www.hollywoodhomestead.com/sibo-solution-resources/

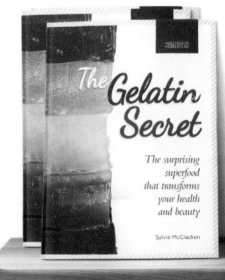

18 Supplements

SIBO WREAKS HAVOC ON YOUR ENTIRE BODY, NOT JUST YOUR GUT. TO HELP YOUR BODY BEAT OFF THE BACTERIA, OVERCOME SYMPTOMS, AND HEAL YOUR GUT, SUPPLEMENTS CAN GO A LONG WAY. HERE ARE SOME OF THE SUPPLEMENTS YOU MAY WANT TO CONSIDER AS PART OF YOUR SIBO TREATMENT. YOU CAN FIND WHERE TO BUY THEM ON OUR RESOURCE PAGE HERE WWW.HOLLYWOODHOMESTEAD.COM/ SIBO-SOLUTION-RESOURCES/

Remember that I am not a doctor and this information isn't intended to be used as medical advice. Always consult with your doctor before taking any supplements.

SUPPLEMENTS FOR TREATING SIBO

When traditional antibiotics failed me, I decided to attack SIBO with a hardcore course of herbal antibiotics. I took ALL of these antibiotics while also doing the elemental diet. Read the chapter about herbal antibiotics on page 40 to learn more about how they work.

- **Allimed (Allicin) 450mg (herbal antibiotic):**
  1–2 capsule 3× per day for a total of 14 days; start with 1 cap 3× per day and on day 3 increase to 2 caps 3× per day

- **Berberine Complex (herbal antibiotic):**
  2–3 capsules 3× per day for a total of 14 days; start with 2 caps 3× per day and on day 3 increase to 3 caps 3× per day

- **Neem Plus (herbal antibiotic):**
  1 capsule 3× per day for a total of 14 days

- **Interfase plus from Klaire Labs (biofilm disruptor):**
  2 capsules 3× per day for a total of 14 days

You can find where to buy these supplements on our resource page here www.hollywoodhomestead.com/sibo-solution-resources/. There is also a discount code for Allimed there too!

> "As a previous SIBO sufferer I was quite knowledgeable about the whole routine. However, this book was the most comprehensive and up to date SIBO resource that I have found online. It was very helpful to see other people's breath test result & to have them explained properly (the doctors never have time to go into so much detail). It was great to have so much info on the different protocols. I am now on my second round of elimination diet with herbal antibiotics & I cannot WAIT to get retested at the end of it. "

> — **SORANA URDAREANU,** ROMANIA

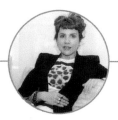

SUPPLEMENTS FOR FIXING NUTRIENT DEFICIENCIES

Your small intestine is the part of your GI system which is responsible for absorbing nutrients into your body. If your small intestine is damaged from SIBO, then you won't be able to absorb nutrients well and can suffer from deficiencies. The bacteria in your gut can also interfere with bile salts, which are important for fat absorption. If you can't absorb fat, then you can end up deficient in the fat soluble vitamins A, D, and E. Finally, bacteria in your gut can consume B_{12}. For these reasons, you might want to consider supplementing during SIBO treatment.

The truth is, until you eliminate SIBO it will be difficult to reverse micronutrient deficiencies. If resources are limited, I would focus on SIBO first and then worry about what deficiencies you have and how to best address them under the care of your doctor.

If money is no object and/or you suspect your micronutrient deficiencies are severe, please see a naturopathic doctor and request that they run a micronutrient panel (I love the Spectracell Labs one) to see what your deficiencies are. This lab test along with a comprehensive CBC (complete blood count) will give you an excellent big picture as to what needs to be addressed more urgently.

If your gut is having trouble absorbing nutrients (which is a given in the case of SIBO), your naturopathic doctor will likely prescribe some custom intramuscular vitamin shots that you can give yourself each week with the specific vitamins you need so you can bypass the gut and still get them in. Note that this is an expensive route to go and unlikely to be covered by insurance, but it's a great option even if you decide to use it as a jump start for only the first few weeks.

Another way to bypass the gut is to use the amazing absorption of your skin! You can ask your doctor about using gut healing supplements that are highly absorbable, such as glutathione.

PROKINETIC SUPPLEMENTS FOR IMPROVING MOTILITY

Read the chapter about motility on page 54 to understand why it is so important for preventing and treating SIBO. You should start taking a prokinetic immediately after you finish your SIBO treatment and continue taking it for 3 months (or as directed by your doctor). If you have an MMC problem, then you may need take prokinetics for the long term to prevent SIBO recurrence. I also took one prokinetic (MotilPro) during treatment, and then added the other two prokinetics after treatment.

- **MotilPro (Pure Encapsulations):** 3 capsules before bed and 3 capsules 1–2 times a day between meals

- **Iberogast:** Take 20 drops before bed or you can use this one with meals

- **Erithromycin:** 50mg before bed (will probably need a prescription for this one as it's a low dose of an antibiotic)

SUPPLEMENTS FOR HEALING THE GUT

There are many things that people can do to heal their gut. However, when you have SIBO, some of the things which are traditionally used for gut healing are way off limits. You have to proceed with caution and check in with your body (or with your lab tests and doctor) to see what works for you and what doesn't. We all have individual tolerances and what works for one might not work for another. A great example of this is gelatin-rich bone broth (which is such an incredible gut healer that I wrote an entire book about it which you can find on the resource page here www.hollywoodhomestead.com/sibo-solution-resources/). But for some SIBO patients, the cartilage (which is high FODMAP) in gelatin can be bothersome. To prevent problems, it is best to make bone broth from marrow bones as they don't contain much cartilage. You can find a recipe for SIBO-friendly bone broth on page 78

Parting Thoughts

IT'S NO DOUBT THAT SIBO, ITS TREATMENT, AND ITS PREVENTION CAN SEEM OVERWHELMING. MY BIGGEST PIECE OF ADVICE IS TO MAKE A PLAN OF ATTACK, COMMIT TO FOLLOWING IT, AND STAY VIGILANT FOR PREVENTION BUT **DON'T LET IT CONSUME YOUR LIFE.**

Your life is about so much more than this condition. Invest in a good doctor, testing, and medicine like your life depends on it (because the quality of your life most definitely does). Use this manual to help guide you along the way. Spend the rest of your time doing things which have nothing to do with SIBO.

Mindset is everything. SIBO is a temporary, acute condition that you absolutely can and will recover from. Set your mind to it, do the work and move on to happier things. ∎

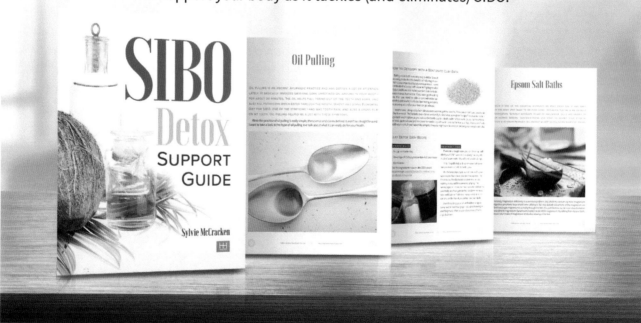

Recipes

BEFORE I WAS DIAGNOSED WITH SIBO, I HAD ALREADY BEEN FOLLOWING A REAL FOOD DIET FOR SEVERAL YEARS. I HAD THOUGHT THAT TRANSITION WAS TOUGH AT TIMES! THE SIBO DIET WAS DIFFERENT THAN ANYTHING I WAS USED TO BECAUSE EVEN A LOT OF HEALTHY THINGS AREN'T GOOD FOR PEOPLE WITH SIBO, SUCH AS GARLIC AND HIGH AMOUNTS OF BROCCOLI AND CAULIFLOWER.

At first, it may seem like The SIBO Diet is super-restrictive and impossible, but I urge you to approach it positively. Don't focus on the things you *can't* eat, but think of all the things you *can* eat. Not only are you helping your body beat and heal from SIBO, but you will probably learn a thing or two about food. If you aren't already used to checking the ingredients on everything you eat, you'll soon be surprised to learn how much sugar, gluten, additives, and other harmful ingredients are lurking in everything from mustard to salad dressings. After a few weeks of vigorous reading of labels, you will really start to rethink all that processed food!

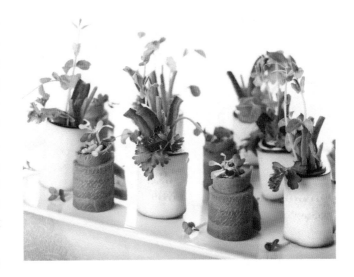

One thing I really want emphasize when it comes to eating on The SIBO Diet is that *ingredient quality matters.*

With meat, you should really strive for pastured, free-range, or wild-caught meat and fish whenever possible. No, this isn't just for the welfare of the animals. When animals have access to the outdoors, they are much healthier than those animals which are cooped up, which means more nutritious meat for us. I am especially a huge advocate of choosing Grass-Fed Pastured beef products because, when cows eat their natural diet of grass instead of being fed grains, their Omega-3:6 ratios are much better. As we talked about on page 71 about healing the gut, Omega-3:6 ratios are really important for people with SIBO in order to reduce inflammation in the gut. You will also want to choose organic and hormone-free meat whenever possible.

Remember to always read the ingredients on food labels before you buy to make sure there aren't any off-limit ingredients or additives in the product. Also keep in mind that small changes can make a big difference to your overall health, like how sea salt is more nutritious than regular table salt.

Most importantly, don't stress. Just do the best you can. The SIBO Diet isn't about perfection. You don't have to completely eliminate all foods which contain FODMAPs. It is about reducing harmful foods to safe limits so bacteria stays under control and your gut can start to heal.

You'll notice that some of the recipes do contain foods on the limited list. Those ingredients are marked with an asterisk (*). The quantities of these foods have been carefully measured so FODMAPs are within safe limits for people with SIBO. However, these are foods that you won't want to have more than one serving of until you know what your body can handle.

I hope these SIBO recipes will serve as a good starting point and you can use them as inspiration to come up with your own recipes. At first it seems restrictive but, once you get the hang of it, it'll be second nature.

Basic Staples

Having SIBO means making some big changes to your meals. No more mashed potatoes for dinner, lattes with lunch, and even most of that healthy salad for lunch is now off limits. You can kind of wrap your head around these big changes, but SIBO also means changes to the small things too. How, for example, do you give flavor to your food when you can't eat garlic? And what about broths for your soup—which are safe to use? Here are a few of the staples which helped me get through The SIBO Diet without feeling deprived and also make meal prep a lot easier.

BEEF BONE BROTH

When I talk about broth, I'm not talking about the broth you buy in the supermarket which comes in a box or can. I'm talking about *real* bone broth which is made from boiling down bones. When you boil down the bones, it releases many nutrients and you get an incredibly healthy, healing liquid which also happens to taste great. I'm such a fan of broth and the gelatin it contains that I wrote a whole book about it, called *The Gelatin Secret*.

For most people, traditional bone broth is one of the best things you can consume and is a great gut healer. For people with SIBO though, broth can be problematic because real broth is typically made from cartilage bones, which are high FODMAP. You can circumvent this problem by using marrow bones (which are low FODMAP) instead of bones containing cartilage. Unfortunately that does mean you will have to specifically buy marrow bones for broth instead of using leftover bones from your roasted chicken dinner. You can get marrow bones at your butcher. Shank bones are particularly good. By the way, you can roast the bones and eat the marrow before using the bones for broth. Roasted marrow tastes awesome.

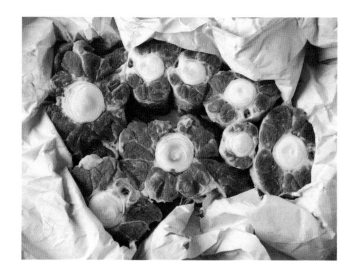

BONE QUALITY

The quality of the bones you use is really important when making broth. Whenever possible, choose beef bones which were Grass-fed and Finished. This means the animals were able to eat their natural diet of grass and not grains like corn. Grass-fed beef has a much better Omega-3:6 ratio and is higher in nutrients. With pork and sheep bones, you will want to look for Free Range products. Always choose Organic and Hormone-Free when you have the chance.

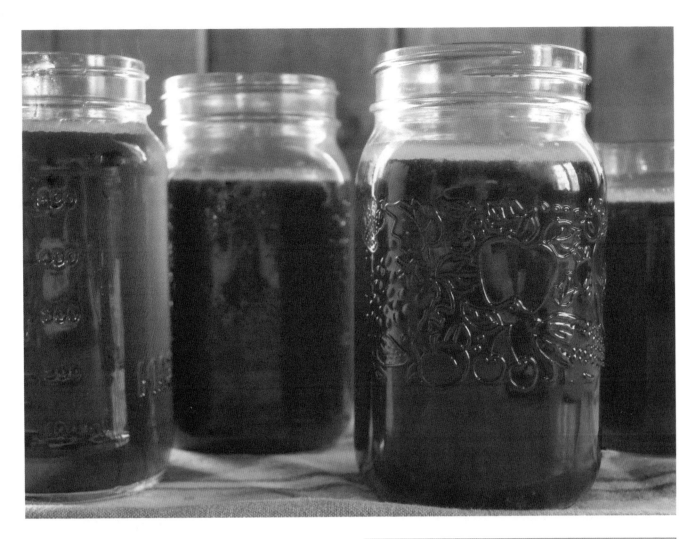

MAKING BONE BROTH

Bone broth is super easy to make. You can use a pressure cooker, slow cooker or just a regular stock pot with the instructions below. You can make a big batch and keep it in the fridge or freezer. You can either simply sip on a cup of warm broth or use as a base for soups or to use in place of water in any savory recipe. If you're in a hurry, you can just make it with the bones, vinegar and water and save the seasoning for later when you're ready to drink the broth or use it in a recipe for more flexibility.

You may be wondering why vinegar is included in this recipe. It's an essential ingredient that will help pull the minerals out of the bones while your stock is simmering in the pot over a long period of time. This recipe for beef bone broth can easily be doubled or even tripled if your soup pot is big enough!

"Last year I was diagnosed with SIBO and received treatment with antibiotics. After the treatment I had a very severe allergic reaction to probiotics that the gastroenterologist prescribed. A clear indication of a very leaky gut. I purchased your book right after that. I read it and started making and consuming broth every week. I also bought the collagen hydrolysate and take it as often as I can remember. I just recently tested negative for leaky gut. Thank you for your hard work. The book is very comprehensive and fun. Love the recipes!"

1. STOCK POT METHOD

If you don't have a slow cooker or pressure cooker, you can make bone broth with this method.

Yield: 1 ½ quarts | **Total Time: 6 hours**

INGREDIENTS

1 ½ lbs beef marrow bones (about 3 bone sections that are each 4″ in length)

2 ½ qt. water

2 leeks, the soft green tops, cut into chunks*

2 carrots, cut into large chunks

¼ cup apple cider vinegar

1 Tbsp butter

2 tsp salt

1 tsp dried thyme

6 whole black peppercorns

1 large Bay leaf

DIRECTIONS

1   Preheat oven to 350°F

2   Put the beef marrow bones on a small rimmed cookie sheet covered with foil and place on the middle rack of a preheated oven. Roast the bones for 45 minutes until somewhat browned.

3   In a large soup pot add the water and the apple cider vinegar along with the soup bones. Place the pot on high heat until the liquid comes to a boil and then immediately turn the heat down to the point where the liquid is just simmering (somewhere between medium and medium-low).

4   Let the soup stock simmer for 3 hours, adding small amounts of water as necessary to keep the bones covered with liquid. Skim off any foam or fat that rises to the surface.

5   Cut the tough green leafy part off of each leek. This will leave you with a white section at the root end of the leek and a light green section that was the mid-part of the leek. Cut the white part away and reserve it for later use. Slice the light green sections in half lengthwise.

6   Add the cut leek sections, 2 whole carrots (unpeeled and chopped into 3 or 4 pieces), bay leaf, dried thyme, 6 whole peppercorns and sea salt to the stock and continue to simmer for another 2 hours. No longer top up the liquid. You want to have the stock reduced to about 1–1 ½ quarts when you are done for a well-flavored and concentrated beef broth. At this point, some people choose to transfer the stock, bones, etc. over to a large crock pot set on high for the rest of the process. You can even let it simmer in the crock-pot overnight if you want.

7   After a minimum of 2 more hours remove the pot from the heat and let the contents cool down for a bit. When cool enough to handle, discard the bones and strain the liquid through a fine sieve to remove the small bits, veggies and peppercorns. When the strained beef stock has cooled to room temperature, cover and refrigerate it overnight. The fat will solidify on top of the stock by the next morning and you can easily skim it off before using this tasty stock in your favorite soup recipe.

* denotes limited amount—please see yes/no list on page 62

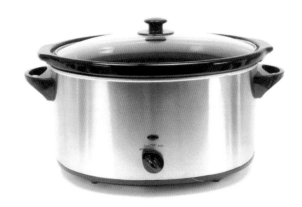

2. SLOW COOKER METHOD

This is the easiest and lowest-maintenance method of making broth.

1   Preheat oven to 350°F

2   Put the beef marrow bones on a small rimmed cookie sheet covered with foil and place on the middle rack of a preheated oven. Roast the bones for 45 minutes until somewhat browned.

3   Turn the slow cooker on to High

4   Add the bones, vegetables, seasonings, and apple cider vinegar to the slow cooker.

5   Add filtered water to the slow cooker until the bones and veggies are covered, leaving about an inch of room at the top.

6   Let it cook for at least 24 hours, ideally 48 or even longer!

7   Once you are ready to harvest your broth, pour it through a strainer into a pot or bowl and allow to cool.

8   Enjoy your broth or store it for later.

9   When the broth cools, you may have a layer of fat on top. Just skim it off.

3. PRESSURE COOKER METHOD

This is the fastest method of making broth but is more hands-on.

1   Preheat oven to 350°F

2   Put the beef marrow bones on a small rimmed cookie sheet covered with foil and place on the middle rack of a preheated oven. Roast the bones for 45 minutes until somewhat browned.

3   Put bones, vegetables, seasonings, and apple cider vinegar into the pressure cooker.

4   Cover with filtered water to ⅔ of the recommended fill point.

5   Close the valve and turn on high and place on a burner on high heat.

6   As soon as the pressure cooker indicates high pressure, turn it to low and cook for 30–40 minutes (not longer).

7   Remove from heat and let the pressure release on its own (about 10 minutes).

8   Strain in a mesh strainer over a bowl or pot.

9   Enjoy the broth! you can reuse your bones for another weaker batch of bone broth if you'd like.

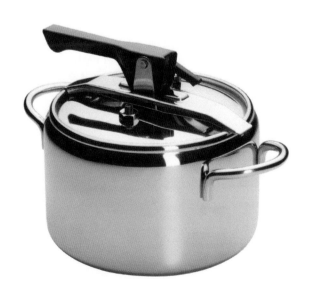

GARLIC INFUSED OLIVE OIL

Giving up garlic, which is high FODMAP is a tough proposition. This recipe is a great way for you to still enjoy the garlic flavor in your cooking without the negative effects. It will be worth the few minutes it takes to make, I promise.
The reason garlic is off limits but garlic infused oil is ok for SIBO sufferers is this: the FODMAPs part of garlic (fructans) is water soluble. They won't leach into the oil. So long as you discard the garlic, garlic infused olive oil is completely okay on The SIBO Diet.

Serves: makes 1 cup | **Total Time: 40 minutes**

INGREDIENTS

1 cup olive oil

1 bulb of garlic separated into individual cloves

DIRECTIONS

1   Peel the garlic by cutting off the ends of the cloves and smashing each clove with the broad side of a flat knife.

2   Heat ¼ cup of the olive oil in a saucepan to the point where it is just simmering and add all of the cloves. Let the cloves simmer in the oil for 5 minutes. They may begin to turn a nice golden color but watch them closely. You don't want the oil to become too hot as it will begin to burn the cloves and this could make the end result bitter. Overheating the oil will also damage it as olive oil has a lower smoke point so keep an eye on it.

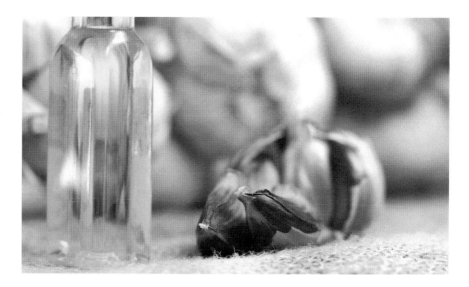

3   Now add the remaining oil and adjust the heat to bring the oil back up to the simmering point. You want to see only a few small bubbles around the cloves. Simmer this way for 15 minutes.

4   Remove from the heat and strain the oil through a fine sieve lined with a few layers of cheesecloth. Discard the garlic cloves.

5   Inspect the strained oil to make sure that every spec of garlic has been removed. If you see small particle of garlic in the oil repeat the straining process using a few more layers of clean cheesecloth.

6   Once the garlic infused olive oil has cooled, store it in the fridge in a sterilized glass jar with a tight fitting lid.

HOMEMADE YOGURT

Simple to make, homemade yogurt not only tastes better than store bought yogurt, it is also much more economical. The list of uses for yogurt is lengthy. It can be the base of a healthy and nutritious breakfast, served up with fresh fruit for a snack, whipped into a tangy salad dressing and a whole lot more.

Many people who eat a lot of yogurt own a yogurt maker, but don't despair if you don't have one. I describe a few, super-easy ways to make yogurt without a lot of fancy equipment. So here's a list of the things you'll need to make your first batch of homemade yogurt (without a yogurt maker):

- Candy thermometer

- Stainless steel or cast iron enamelled pot **or** a thermos **or** a large glass jar (these will be used as an incubator for your yogurt)

- Stainless steel whisk and a ladle

- Cheesecloth for straining if you want a thicker yogurt consistency—as in Greek-style yogurt

- Mason jars for storing yogurt in the fridge

Serves: makes 2 quarts yogurt | **Total Time: 10 minutes, incubation period—24 hours**

*Even though your yogurt may be done faster, always let it ferment for 24–37 hours before putting it in the fridge. This is important for SIBO patients so they get the right levels of healthy bacteria.

INGREDIENTS

2 qt whole milk, (preferably raw, second best is grass fed, third best is simply organic)

½ cup yogurt or a package of dried yogurt culture (find out where to buy on our resource page here www.hollywoodhomestead.com/sibo-solution-resources/)

DIRECTIONS

1   Sterilize the equipment you will be using. You can do this by setting your dishwasher to the "sanitize" setting or by using the boiling water bath method.

2   Pour the milk into a pot with the candy thermometer attached to the side making sure the bottom of the thermometer isn't touching the bottom of the pot.

3   Heat the milk over a burner turned to medium-high until the milk reaches the boiling point (180°F), stirring constantly.

4   Immediately remove from heat and let the milk cool down to 110–115°F.

5   If you are using fresh yogurt as a culture, mix a little of the warm milk into the yogurt to thin it out and then mix the thinned yogurt into the warm milk in the large pot.

6   If you are using a powdered culture, follow the manufacturer's directions when adding the powder to the warmed milk in the pot.

7   The directions for making yogurt are identical up to this point. Read on for descriptions of three different methods you can use at home (without a yogurt maker).

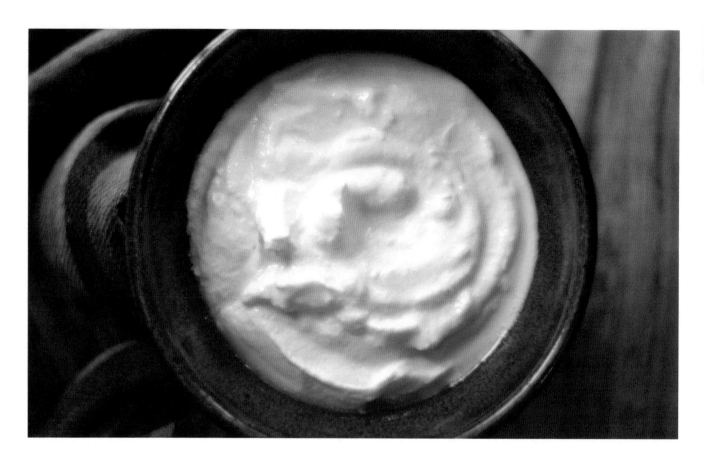

METHOD 1

If you own a heavy enameled cast iron pot this is the way to go. If you use it for the first part of the process described above the cast iron will be nice and warm when you add the yogurt or powdered culture to the milk. Simply turn the light on in your unheated oven. Cover the pot with its cast iron lid and place the pot in the oven close to the side where the oven light is located. The heat from the light bulb will keep the oven warm. Leave the pot without disturbing it for at least four hours or more. You can take it out of the oven after that, but let it ferment for 24–37 hours before you put it in the fridge. I usually do my yogurt prep just before bedtime, leave everything in the oven overnight and always have a good result in the morning. What could be easier than that!

METHOD 2

This is how I used to make yogurt before I owned a cast iron pot. Place the milk mixture in a large sterilized glass jar with a tight fitting lid. Wrap a small quilt, comforter or child's sleeping bag around the jar and put it on top of your fridge. The motor of the plugged in fridge lets off a bit of heat and if you place the wrapped up jar towards the back of top of the fridge your jar will stay nice and warm. Again, leave it for 24–37 hours.

METHOD 3

An insulated thermos makes a great incubator too. Simply pre-heat the interior by filling the thermos up with really hot tap water and set it aside until you are ready for it.

*Note: *If you find your yogurt is thinner than you like simply place the yogurt in a fine sieve, lined with a few layers of cheesecloth and place the sieve over a deep bowl. Let the yogurt drain out until it thickens into the required consistency.*

SAUSAGE SPICE BLENDS

Having a couple spice blends on hand that you can prep ahead of time is a great tool to have when you're on The SIBO Diet. That way you know you have a couple of spice blends you can use when cooking without having to check your yes/no list. You can even make one up to carry in your purse if you plan to eat out and ask the waiter to keep your food unseasoned (like a simple grilled meat) and season it yourself.

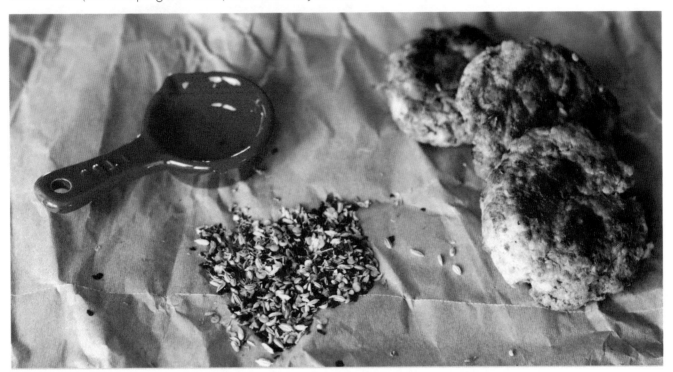

SPICY ITALIAN SAUSAGE SPICE BLEND

This is the spice blend used for the sausage recipe on page <u>102</u> but it's also a great spice blend to have on hand for other foods you'd like to season.

Serves: 4 | **Total time: 3 minutes**

INGREDIENTS

1 Tbsp dried oregano

1 tsp crushed red pepper flakes

1 tsp fennel seed

1–2 tsp sea salt

1 tsp fresh cracked black pepper

⅛ tsp cayenne pepper, or more to taste

DIRECTIONS

1 Combine spices to create the spice blend. Double, triple or quadruple the recipe to make bigger batches.

2 Store in a glass jar or reuse a salt shaker.

3 Use on anything you want!

Savory Sage Spice Blend

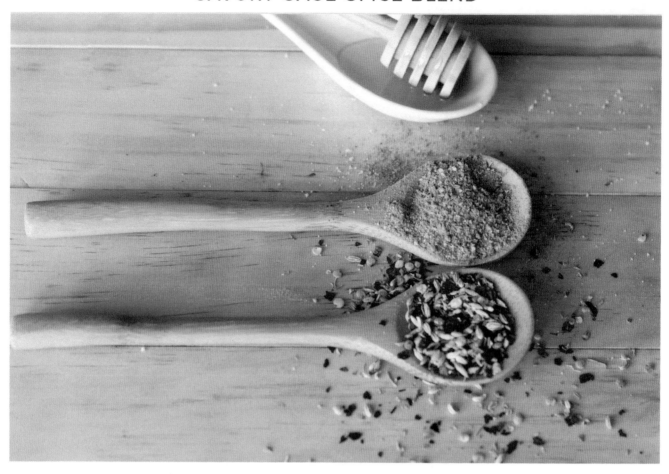

Serves: 4 | **Total Time: 3 minutes**

INGREDIENTS

1 tsp rubbed sage

1 tsp marjoram

½ tsp sea salt

⅛ tsp ground cinnamon

⅛ tsp ground nutmeg

DIRECTIONS

1. Combine spices to create the spice blend. Double, triple or quadruple the recipe to make bigger batches.

2. Store in a glass jar or reuse a salt shaker.

3. Use on anything you want!

Lemon Ginger Vinaigrette Dressing

Having a salad dressing on hand in the fridge, especially if you're used to buying store bought salad dressings, can be helpful for when you want to make a quick salad and have something interesting to dress it with. This very simple dressing is one of my favorites. Keep in mind it won't store as long as store bought dressings loaded with preservatives so I'd recommend making this recipe once every 10 days or so and keeping it refrigerated.

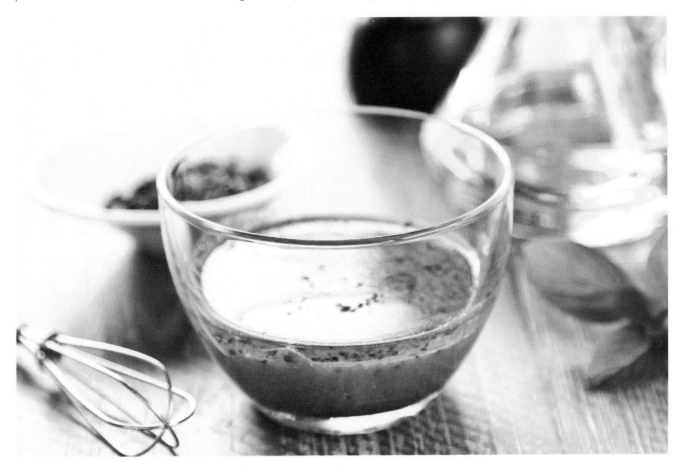

Serves: 6–8 | **Total Time: 5 minutes**

INGREDIENTS

¼ cup olive oil

¼ cup fresh lemon juice

1 Tbsp fresh grated (or finely chopped) ginger

1 tsp dried oregano

Pinch of salt

DIRECTIONS

1 Combine all the ingredients in a small bowl or salad dressing container.

2 If in a bowl whisk the ingredients together until they are well blended. If using a salad dressing container shake vigorously until the ingredients are blended together.

3 Serve over your favorite salad and enjoy.

Breakfast

If you're used to having tons of grains like cereals and muffins for breakfast, then breakfast on The SIBO Diet will be a bit of a change of pace. If you're in a hurry you can always do something simple like scrambled eggs and be on your way but, if you have a little time, you can make a frittata or some sausage patties to eat throughout the week or freeze for later. Here are some ideas to get you started.

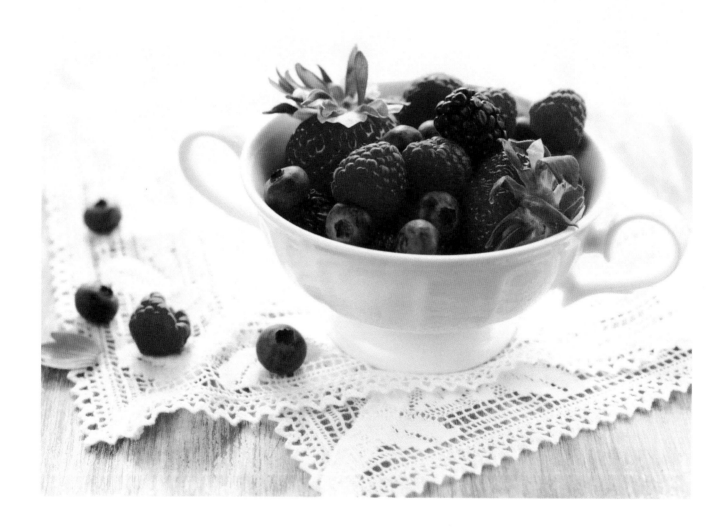

BANANA NUT MUFFINS

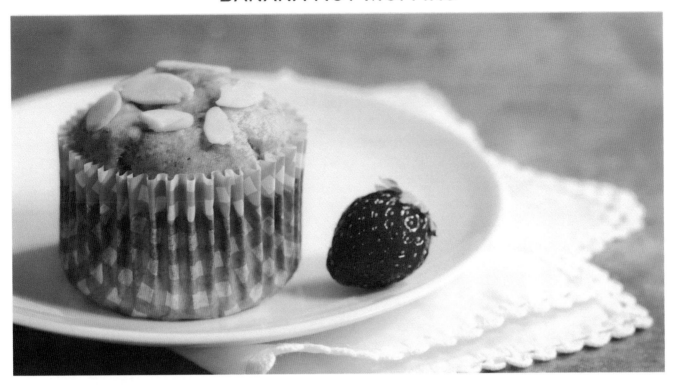

Serves: 1 | **Total Time: 25 minutes**

This is a perfect recipe for using up bananas that are overripe and passed their prime. Ready in twenty five minutes, this version of banana bread serves one. You simply mix the ingredients up, pop it in the oven and presto; a nice warm and moist banana bread to start the day.

INGREDIENTS

½ Banana, mashed

1 Egg, beaten

2 Tbsp almond flour*

1 Tbsp coconut flour*

1 Tbsp honey*

1 Tbsp almond butter

1 tsp coconut oil

¼ tsp vanilla

¼ tsp baking soda

Pinch of Cinnamon

Pinch of Salt

DIRECTIONS

1 Pre-heat oven to 350 degrees

2 Whisk egg in a small bowl.

3 Combine with mashed banana, honey, coconut oil & vanilla in a small bowl.

4 Add the almond flour, coconut flour, baking soda, cinnamon & salt. Mix until all ingredients are well combined.

5 Spoon the batter into a large-sized, oiled muffin tin.

6 Bake on the middle rack of the pre-heated oven for 20 minutes.

You can double the recipe for two beautiful banana nut muffins.

* denotes limited amount—please see yes/no list on page 62

Banana Nut Smoothie

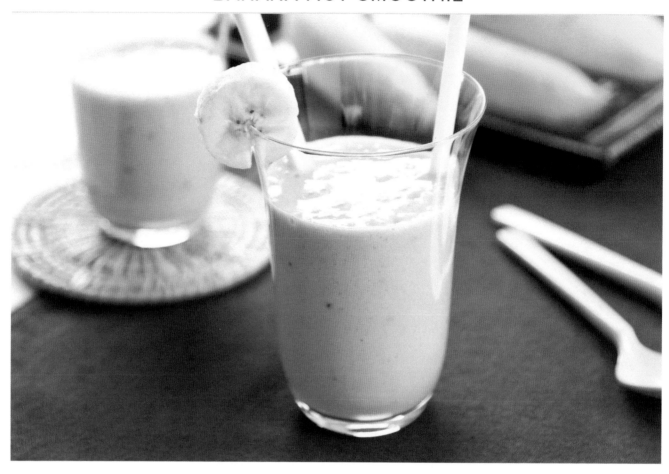

Serves: 2 | **Total Time: 3 minutes**

INGREDIENTS

2 bananas, frozen

½ cup Homemade Yogurt (see recipe on page 83)

½ cup coconut milk*

½ cup coconut water

2 Tbsp almond butter*

2 Tbsp honey*

2 or 3 ice cubes

DIRECTIONS

1   Place all the ingredients in a blender and process on high speed for one minute until everything is well blended.

2   Enjoy!

* denotes limited amount—please see yes/no list on page 62

Green Smoothie

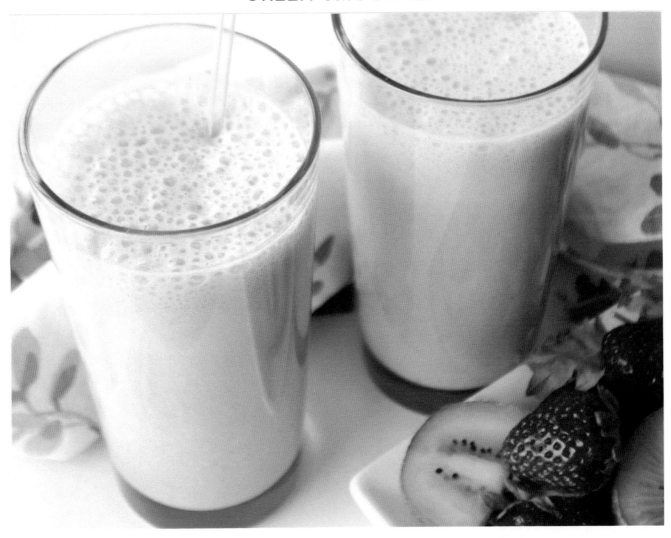

Serves: 2 | **Total Time: 3 minutes**

INGREDIENTS

1 banana, frozen and cut into chunks

2 cups baby kale leaves or spinach leaves

½ cup strawberries, frozen

1 kiwi, peeled

¾ cup cold water (or ½ cup water and 2 or 3 ice cubes)

½ cup coconut milk*

½ cup Homemade Yogurt (see recipe on page 83)

2–3 Tbsp. honey*

DIRECTIONS

1   Place all the ingredients in a blender and process on high speed for one minute until everything is well blended and the kale leaves are completely incorporated into the smoothie.

* denotes limited amount—please see yes/no list on page 62

Breakfast Bowl

I make a breakfast bowl when I want to change it up a bit in the morning. I've used ground beef in this bowl but you could easily substitute any ground meat you have on hand. There's also a wide range of spice and herb options that work equally well. You could opt for a curry flavored breakfast bowl or throw in oregano and basil for an Italian version of this versatile dish. If I have leftover Roasted Root Vegetables (from the recipe on page 110) from the night before I'll use those instead of the cooked squash. Tasty and filling, a breakfast bowl is the perfect way to fuel your body for the busy day that lies ahead.

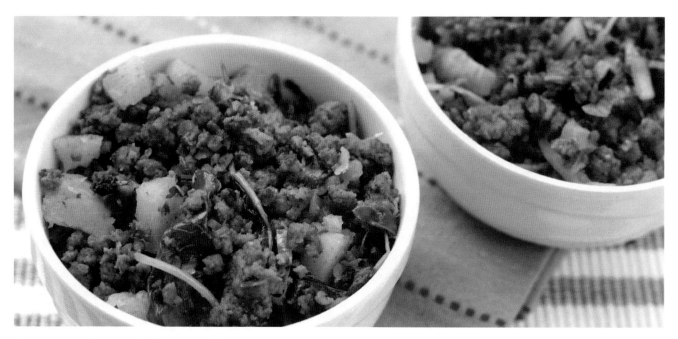

Serves: 2 | **Total Time: 15 minutes**

INGREDIENTS

½ lb Ground Beef

2 cups kale or spinach leaves, shredded & tightly packed

½ Leek, sliced thinly*

½ cup butternut squash, cooked*

¼ cup almond milk

1 Tbsp fresh thyme leaves

2 tsp olive oil

Salt & pepper to taste

DIRECTIONS

1   In a skillet heated to medium-, sauté the sliced leek in olive oil until it softens.

2   Add the ground beef to the skillet and continue to stir and cook the beef/leek mixture until the beef is browned and cooked through.

3   While continuing to stir the mixture, add the cooked squash, almond milk and thyme leaves.

4   When all the ingredients are heated through, adjust the seasonings with salt & pepper, divide into two bowls and serve.

* denotes limited amount—please see yes/no list on page 62

LEEK & ROASTED RED PEPPER FRITTATA

It's hard to beat eggs in the morning. When served in a frittata with roasted red peppers, leeks and an aged cheddar cheese, the end result is a scrumptious combo your family will love even if they are not eating The SIBO Diet.

Serves: 4 | **Total Time: 25 minutes**

INGREDIENTS

8 Eggs, whisked

1 Red pepper, roasted and cut into small dice

2 Leeks, white part only—thinly sliced*

½ cup aged cheddar cheese, grated (use white cheese)*

1 Tbsp olive oil

1 tsp basil (or 1 Tbsp fresh leaves chopped finely)

¼ tsp sea salt

Grinding of pepper

DIRECTIONS

1   Roast the pepper. To do this, first remove the seeds and membrane and then cut it into flat pieces. Put the pieces skin side up on a cookie sheet that has been lightly oiled with your cooking fat of choice. Place the cookie sheet under the broiler in your oven and leave the peppers pieces there until they are charred. Once blackened, remove them from the oven and let the peppers cool. You will find the charred skins pull off easily and the resulting roasted pepper pieces will have a deep and mellow flavor.

2   Sauté the sliced leeks in olive oil in a small sized skillet placed over medium-high heat.

3   Add the roasted red pepper and spread the leek and pepper mixture evenly over the bottom of the skillet.

4   Pour the whisked eggs into the skillet slowly so the leek/pepper mixture remains evenly dispersed around the bottom of the skillet.

5   Turn the heat down to medium and when the egg begins to firm up on the bottom, gently lift the sides of the firming egg so that the liquid egg on top runs underneath the firmed up egg. Lift various areas around the edge and repeat the process. When the egg is almost completely firm sprinkle the cheddar cheese over the top and pop the skillet under the broiler in the oven to melt the cheese.

6   When the cheese is bubbling and slightly browned remove the frittata from the oven and serve.

* denotes limited amount—please see yes/no list on page 62

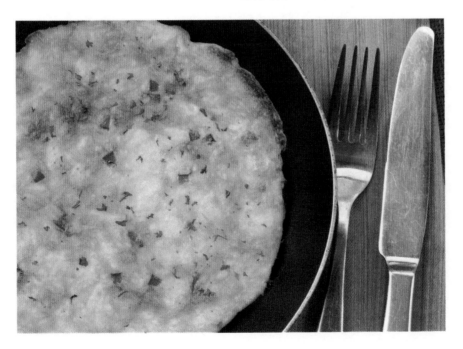

Main Courses

The great thing about The SIBO Diet is that protein (other than processed stuff with added sugars like many brands of bacon) isn't limited. This gives you a ton of flexibility when it comes to creating main courses.

Remember, as we discussed on page 102, the quality of the meat, poultry, eggs and fish is important. Choose pasture-raised, free-range, wild-caught and organic whenever possible.

Beef

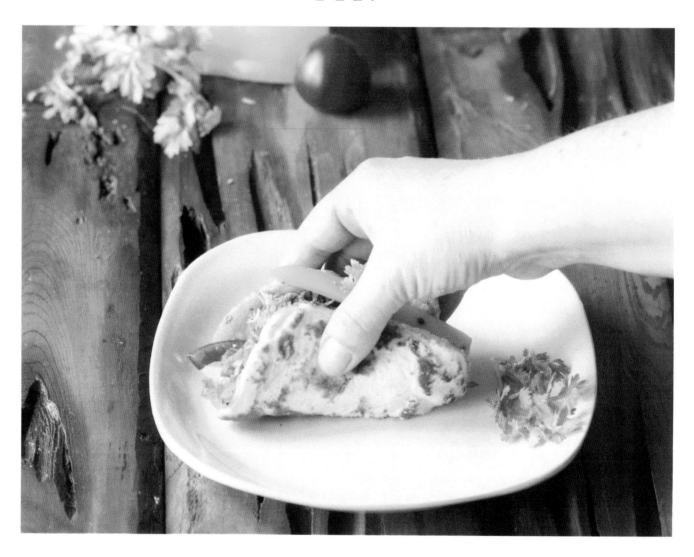

BEEF CARNITAS WITH COCONUT FLOUR TORTILLAS

Serves: 2 | **Total Time: 8 hours**

INGREDIENTS

Beef Carnitas

2 cups water

1 (1 lb) sirloin steak

1 bell pepper, sliced

1 tsp paprika

1 tsp cumin

½ tsp cayenne

1 tsp chili powder

1 tsp salt

For the Tortillas

5 egg whites

¼ cup coconut flour*

¼ cup unsweetened almond
  milk (without thickeners)*

1 tsp cumin

½ tsp chili powder

¼ tsp sea salt

coconut oil

Optional Additional Toppings:

Shredded Cheese*

Broccoli*

Shredded Napa Cabbage

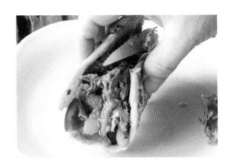

DIRECTIONS

1 Mix together the paprika, cumin, cayenne, chili powder, and salt in small bowl to make a spice rub for the beef.

2 Rub the spice rub mixture all over the sirloin steak, massaging it into the meat.

3 Place the steak in the slow cooker then pour the water around it.

4 Turn the slow cooker on low for 8 hours.

5 After 8 hours, remove and shred the beef with two forks. Remove the bones and place the meat back into the juices until ready to serve.

For the Tortillas (makes 4 tortillas)

1 Add the egg whites, coconut flour, almond milk, cumin, chili powder and salt to a blender or food processor.

2 Process until well combined. It will be thin.

3 Allow the batter to sit for 5–7 minutes.

4 Place a small nonstick skillet over medium heat.

5 Add the coconut oil and move the pan around to make sure it covers the entire surface.

6 Using a ladle, add ¼ of the mixture to the hot skillet.

7 Lift it up and move it around to spread the batter around in a circle in the skillet.

8 Cook for 2–3 minutes on one side, until the exposed side is no longer shiny.

9 Flip carefully, using a large spatula.

10 Cook another 1–2 minutes, or until browned.

11 Remove, and set aside.

12 Repeat with remaining batter to make 4 tortillas.

13 Do not place them on top of each other; they will stick! A paper towel lined plate works best.

To Assemble:

1 Spoon the beef into the tortillas. Add the bell peppers, and other veggies if desired.

* denotes limited amount—please see yes/no list on page <u>62</u>

Spaghetti & Meatballs: Paleo Style

Serves: 4 (32 small meatballs) | **Total Time: 45 minutes**

INGREDIENTS

1 lb Italian Spiced Turkey Sausage
(see recipe on page 102)

12 ripe plum tomatoes

2 leeks (white part only), sliced thinly*

6 Tbsp fresh basil

4 Tbsp flat leaf parsley

4 Tbsp fresh oregano leaves

2 Tbsp butter

1 Tbsp olive oil

Salt & pepper to taste

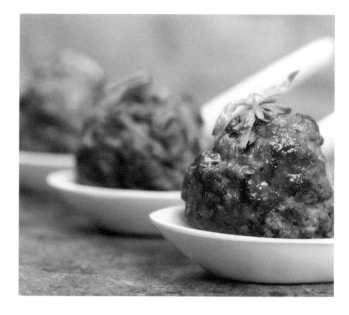

DIRECTIONS

1 Preheat oven to 350 degrees

2 Make small meatballs using the turkey sausage by rolling about a tablespoon of the sausage meat between the palms of your hands. One pound of sausage meat should make 32 small meatballs. Rubbing a scant amount of oil on your palms will keep the meat from sticking.

3 Brush rimmed cookie sheet with a small amount of oil, or line it with parchment paper. Place meatballs on the cookie sheet. Bake meatballs for 20 minutes.

4 Chop the flat leaf parsley, snip the oregano leaves off of the stems, chiffonade the basil into thin strips and set aside.

5 Heat the butter and the olive oil in a saucepan over medium-high heat. When the oil/melted butter mixture is very hot add the leeks. Sauté for three or four minutes.

6 Meanwhile, cut the end out of each tomato and chop them all coarsely. When the leeks have softened and start becoming translucent, add the chopped tomatoes to them.

7 Bring the leek and tomato mixture until they start simmering and then lower the heat to a point where the mixture continues to cook at a bare simmer. Cook for 15 minutes, stirring occasionally.

8 Add the parsley, oregano and 2 tbsp of the basil to the sauce and continue to simmer for another 5 minutes.

9 The meatballs should be just coming out of the oven now. You can add them right into the tomato sauce and simmer for another 5 minutes. Adjust the seasoning by adding salt & pepper to suit your taste buds. Serve over zucchini noodles (recipe follows) and garnish with reserved basil.

QUICK ZUCCHINI NOODLES

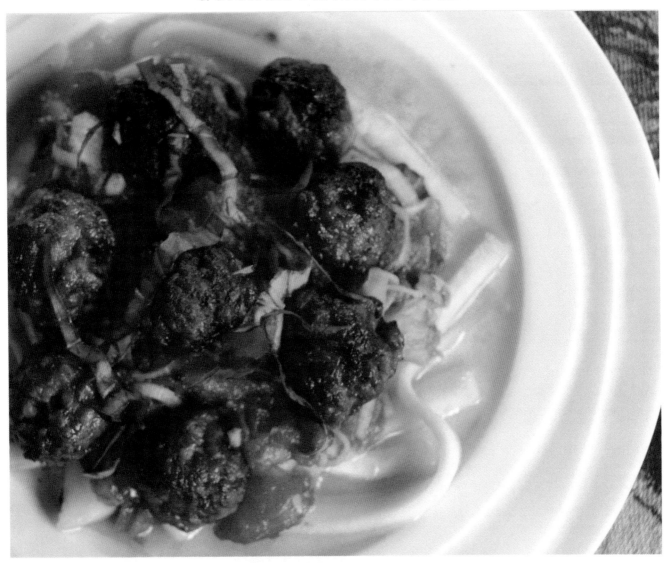

4 small yellow zucchini*

1 Tbsp butter

salt & pepper

1 Cut the zucchini lengthwise into very thin slices

2 Now carefully cut each slice into flat "noodles" lengthwise.

3 Melt the butter in a medium sized frying pan place over a burner set to medium high

4 When the butter has melted and is hot add the zucchini noodles all at once. Sauté until the noodles become somewhat soft and are heated through. This won't take very long; about 4 or 5 minutes at most.

5 Adjust the seasoning with salt and pepper to taste.

* denotes limited amount—please see yes/no list on page 62

BEEF & VEGGIE SOUP

I've used carrots, cabbage, leeks and broccoli in this recipe but really you can use whatever veggies you have on hand. Just make sure you pay attention to the amounts you use according to the foods allowed list so you can accurately figure out the number of portions you've made.

Serves: 4 | **Total Time: 1.5 hours**

INGREDIENTS

1 lb marinating beef steak cut into 1 inch cubes

1 qt Beef Bone Broth (recipe on page 78)

4 cups shredded cabbage*

2 cups broccoli, cut into small pieces*

2 Leeks, white part only, sliced thinly*

2 medium size carrots, finely diced

2 Tbsp fresh thyme leaves

1 Tbsp butter

1 Tbsp olive oil

1 bay leaf

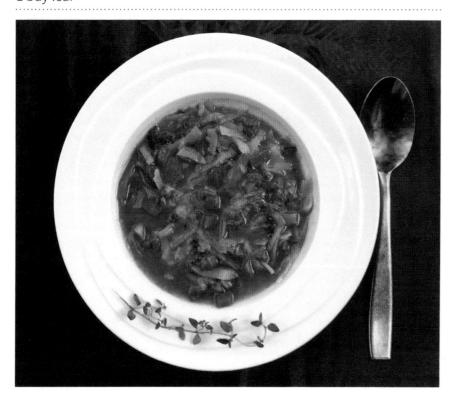

DIRECTIONS

1   Heat butter and olive oil in large soup pot over medium high heat.

2   Add leeks and sauté for 1 minute before adding the cubed beef. Sauté the leek and beef mixture for 2 more minutes until the meat begins to brown.

3   Add the diced carrots and shredded cabbage to the pot followed by the beef broth and bay leaf. Once the soup starts to boil, turn down the heat and let the soup simmer for about 45 minutes before adding the broccoli and fresh thyme.

4   Simmer for another 15 minutes then correct the seasoning by adding salt and pepper if needed.

* denotes limited amount—please see yes/no list on page 62

BEEF AND BROCCOLI

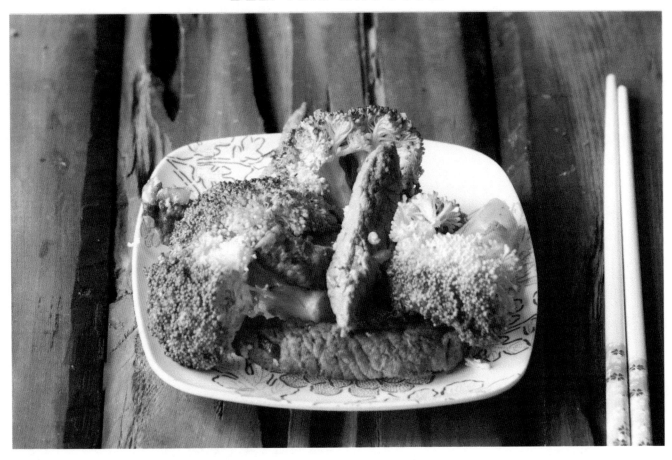

Serves: 2 | **Total Time: 20 minutes**

INGREDIENTS

1 round steak, cut into strips

1 cup broccoli, cut into florets (½ each serving)*

1 orange

1 Tbsp apple cider vinegar

½ inch ginger, minced

sea salt and black pepper, to taste

coconut oil

DIRECTIONS

1 Add the coconut oil to a medium skillet and heat on medium-high.

2 Add the steak strips to the hot skillet and sauté for 3–4 minutes.

3 Add the broccoli, juice from the orange, apple cider, and ginger.

4 Season with salt and pepper.

5 Continue to sauté until the steak is cooked to desired doneness.

* denotes limited amount—please see yes/no list on page 62

YELLOW ZUCCHINI PASTA WITH TURKEY MEATBALLS

Serves: 2 | **Total Time: 25 minutes**

INGREDIENTS

½ lb ground turkey

2 yellow zucchini

3 tomatoes, quartered

1 egg

1 Tbsp almond meal*

1 Tbsp oregano

4–5 basil leaves

½ tsp salt

olive oil

salt and pepper, to taste

DIRECTIONS

1 In a medium mixing bowl, add the turkey, almond meal, turkey, oregano, and ½ tsp. salt.

2 Use your hands to mix well.

3 Form meatballs (about 6) and set aside.

4 Heat a medium skillet over medium-high heat. Add a drizzle of coconut or olive oil.

5 Place the meatballs in the hot skillet and cook 3–5 minutes on each side, turning frequently to brown all sides until cooked through. Remove to heat and set aside.

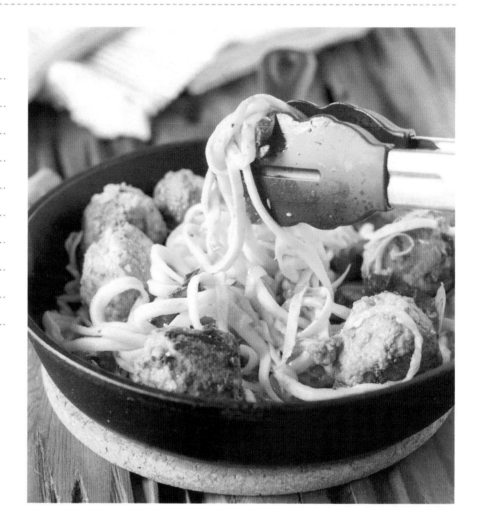

6 Use a spiralizer to create the yellow zucchini pasta. Set aside.

7 Add a drizzle of olive oil or coconut oil to the same pan the meatballs were cooked in.

8 Add the yellow zucchini pasta and quartered tomatoes. Season with salt.

9 Sauté the "noodles" until warmed through.

10 Serve with meatballs and garnish of fresh basil.

* denotes limited amount—please see yes/no list on page 62

LEMON DIJON CHICKEN

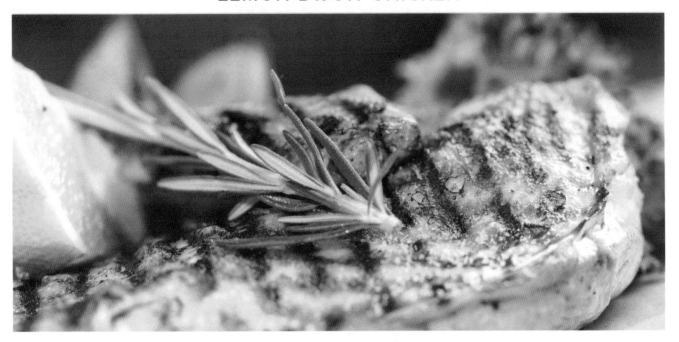

This recipe comes together quickly and is a perfect choice when you need a meal in a hurry. You could also double the recipe and use the leftovers for a chicken salad for the next day.

Serves: 2 | **Total Time: 25 minutes**

INGREDIENTS

2 chicken breasts

¼ cup chicken broth or white wine

2 Tbsp dijon mustard

2 Tbsp mayonnaise

grinding of pepper

5 or 6 sprigs of fresh thyme

Juice and rind (grated) from ½ lemon

DIRECTIONS

1 Preheat oven to 350°F

2 Rub each chicken breast with 1 Tbsp of dijon mustard on both sides and place side by side in a small casserole dish. Grind pepper over them.

3 Sprinkle the zest from the lemon over the chicken breast and drizzle the juice from the lemon over top of everything

4 Top the chicken breasts with the sprigs of fresh thyme.

5 Carefully pour the chicken stock (or wine) around the outside edges of the chicken breasts.

6 Place the casserole on the middle rack of the preheated oven and bake for 20 minutes or until the internal temperature of the chicken reaches 165 degrees.

7 Remove the chicken. Put it on a plate and drain off the juices. Collect the juices in a bowl. You may need to strain the juices to get out the small bits of chicken.

8 Add 2 tbsp. of mayonnaise to the strained juices and whisk together to make a smooth sauce. Serve in a small dish beside the chicken.

HOMEMADE ITALIAN SPICED TURKEY SAUSAGE

Yield: 3 lbs of sausage meat | **Prep Time: 5 minutes**

INGREDIENTS

3 lbs ground turkey

3 Tbsp red wine vinegar

1 Tbsp black pepper

1 Tbsp dried parsley
(3 tbsp fresh parsley leaves)

1 Tbsp dried basil
(3 tbsp fresh basil leaves)

1 Tbsp oregano
(3 tbsp fresh oregano)

1 Tbsp ground fennel

2 tsp paprika

2 tsp crushed red pepper flakes

2 tsp salt

1 tsp dried thyme
(1 tbsp fresh Thyme)

¼ tsp pure stevia
(optional—traditional Italian sausage has just a hint of sweetness and stevia in small amounts is allowed on The SIBO Diet but if you prefer to stick to 100% whole foods you can definitely leave it out)

You will notice I've provided measurements for both dried and fresh herbs. Use three times the amount of fresh herb when substituting fresh herbs for dried herbs; that's the general rule of thumb. I would recommend using the dried herbs if you are planning on freezing the sausage meat.

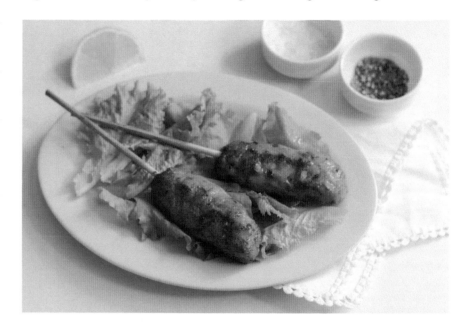

DIRECTIONS

1 Place the ground turkey into a large bowl and simply add all of the ingredients listed above. Mix everything together until the spices are evenly distributed throughout the ground meat.

2 Wrap the sausage mixture up tightly in plastic wrap and refrigerate for 12 hours. This gives the flavors a chance to blend and develop before using in your favorite recipes or you can simply freeze for later use.

SERVING SUGGESTION

1 Pre-heat oven to 400°F.

2 For a quick meal form egg-shaped balls of meat and insert a skewer into the centre of each. Place turkey skewers on a parchment lined cookie sheet and bake in the pre-heated oven for about half an hour. The meat should be nicely browned and slightly crispy on the outside when the turkey skewers are done.

Coconut Crusted Chicken with Spinach Salad

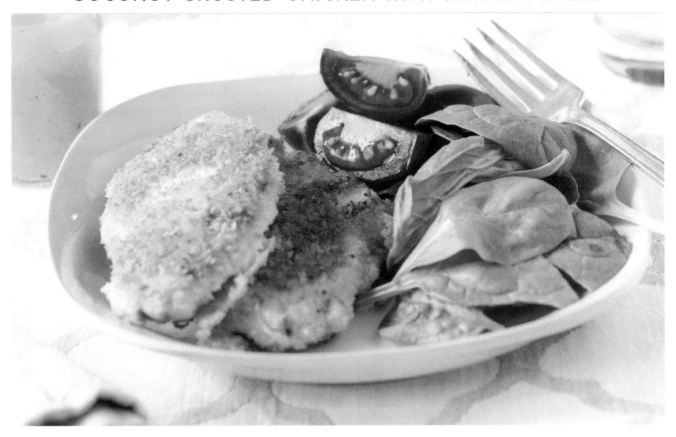

Serves: 1 | **Total Time: 20 minutes**

INGREDIENTS

1–2 chicken fillets

1 egg, beaten

13 spinach leaves

1 tomato, quartered

2 Tbsp apple cider vinegar

1 Tbsp coconut flour*

1 Tbsp unsweetened
flaked coconut*

½ tsp. clover honey*

drizzle of olive oil

salt and pepper, to taste

coconut oil

DIRECTIONS

1 Allow the chicken fillets to come to room temperature.

2 Place the coconut flour on one plate, coconut flakes on a separate plate, and egg in a bowl. This is your dredging station.

3 Place the chicken fillet in the coconut flour, coating the fillet. Next dip it into the eggs, turning to coat the fillet. Finally, put it in the coconut flakes, turning to coat the fillet.

4 Add the coconut oil to a skillet over medium heat.

5 Place the coated fillets in the hot skillet and cook for 4–5 minutes on each side or until the fillets are golden brown and cooked through. Set aside.

6 In a small bowl, mix the apple cider vinegar, and honey. Whisk in the olive oil until well combined. Season with salt and pepper.

7 Plate the chicken with the spinach, tomato and dressing on the side.

* denotes limited amount—please see yes/no list on page 62

PECAN HONEY MUSTARD CRUSTED SALMON SALAD

Serves: 2 | **Total Time: 20 minutes**

INGREDIENTS

For Salmon

2 (5oz) salmon fillets

1 ½ Tbsp pecans, chopped finely*

1 Tbsp gluten-free mustard

1 Tbsp clover honey*

Olive oil, for greasing pan

Salt, to taste

For Salad

1 cup arugula, chopped

1 cup spinach, chopped

1 cup carrots, shredded

½ cucumber, chopped

2 Tbsp pomegranate seeds*

1 Tbsp pumpkin seeds, roasted*

For Dressing

1 Tbsp mustard

1 Tbsp white wine vinegar

1 Tbsp olive oil

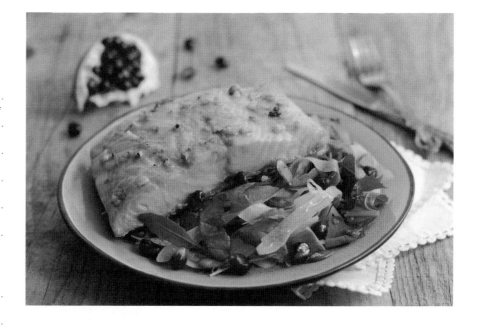

DIRECTIONS

1 Preheat oven to 350°F.

2 Place the salmon on an oiled baking sheet. Season with salt.

3 In a small bowl combine the chopped pecans, mustard, and honey. Mix until a paste forms. Use your hands to cover the top of the salmon filets with the paste, being sure to press down as you go.

4 Place the salmon in the oven and bake for 12–16 minutes, until cooked through and flakes with a fork.

5 While the salmon is cooking combine all the ingredients for the salad in a large mixing bowl.

6 In another small bowl whisk together the ingredients for the dressing. Pour the dressing over the salad ingredients and toss to coat.

7 Once the fish is done remove it from the oven.

8 Divide the salad evenly between two plates. Top with the salmon fillets and serve.

* denotes limited amount—please see yes/no list on page 62

FISH TACOS

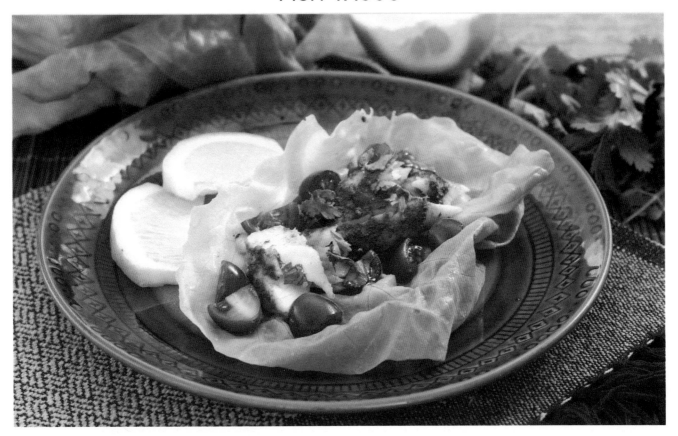

Serves: 2 | **Total Time: 21 minutes**

INGREDIENTS

2 4oz cod filets

10 cherry tomatoes, quartered

4 lettuce leaves
(These will be your tacos;
Boston Lettuce works well)

1 Tbsp olive oil

1 Tbsp fresh parsley, chopped

1 tsp cumin

1 tsp smoked paprika

Salt, to taste

4 lemon wedges, for garnish

DIRECTIONS

1 Preheat oven to 400°F.

2 In a small bowl mix together the cumin and smoked paprika.

3 Place the cod filets in a baking dish. Drizzle the fish with the olive oil. Season with salt to taste. Sprinkle the spice mix over the fish, dividing evenly.

4 Bake in the oven for 13–16 minutes, until the fish is cooked through and flakes with a fork.

5 Remove the fish from the oven. Divide each of the fish filets between the lettuce leaves, making 4 tacos total. Divide the chopped tomatoes between the tacos. Serve with lemon wedges and sprinkle with fresh parsley for garnish.

Shrimp Kabob

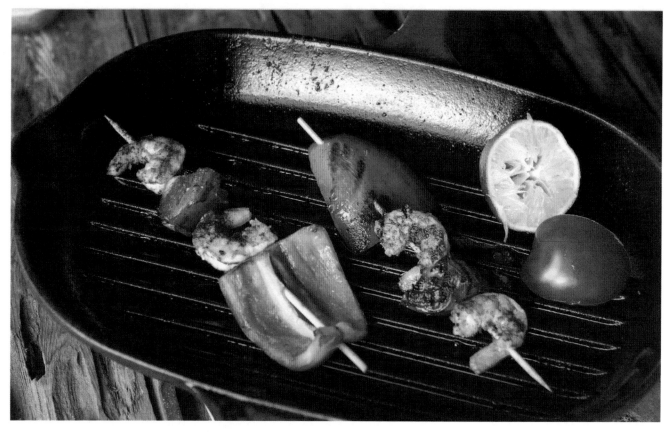

Serves: 2 | **Total Time: 15 minutes**

INGREDIENTS

About 20 shrimp shrimp, peeled and deveined

3 bell pepper, cut into large chunks

3 tomatoes, cut into large chunks

1 tsp chili powder

1 tsp cumin

½ tsp sea salt

Juice from 1 lime

Coconut Oil

4 small bamboo skewers or 2 long skewers

DIRECTIONS

1   Place the shrimp in a small bowl and add the lime juice, chili powder, cumin, and sea salt. Stir to coat. Set aside for 10 minutes.

2   Soak 4 bamboo skewers in water while the shrimp is marinating.

3   Spear a bell pepper, follow by a shrimp, then a tomato, and repeat until skewer is full. Repeat until all the ingredients are used.

4   Heat the coconut oil in a grill pan over medium high heat.

5   Once the oil is melted, place the skewers into the hot pan. Grill 4–5 minutes on each side, or until the shrimp is pink and cooked through.

6   Serve immediately. Enjoy!

Side Dishes

THE MAIN COURSES ON THE SIBO DIET ARE PRETTY EASY, SINCE YOU HAVE SO MANY PROTEIN OPTIONS TO CHOOSE FROM. THE SIDE DISHES ARE WHERE THINGS CAN SOMETIMES GET TRICKY SINCE THE VEGETABLE LIST IS THE ONE THAT IS MUCH MORE RESTRICTIVE IN TERMS OF WHICH VEGETABLES ARE ALLOWED AND WHICH ONES NEED TO BE LIMITED.

Please note the asterisks on these recipes; those are ingredients which have been carefully measured out so that they are compliant with the quantities allowed on The SIBO Diet. Use these side dish recipes as starting points to create your own recipes as well!

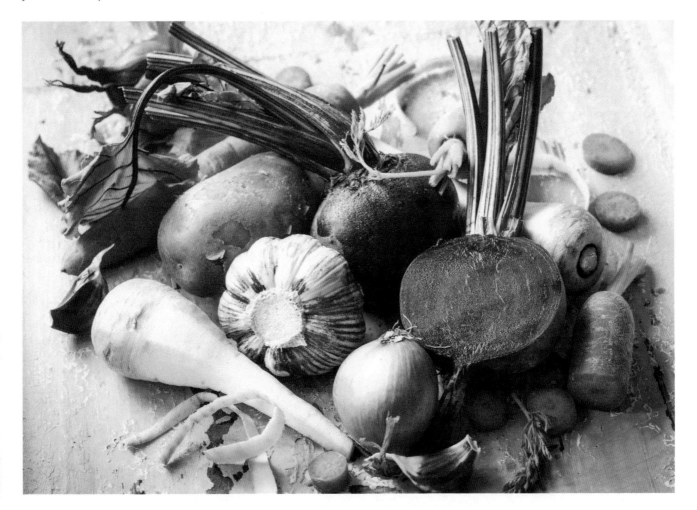

Honey Ginger Carrots

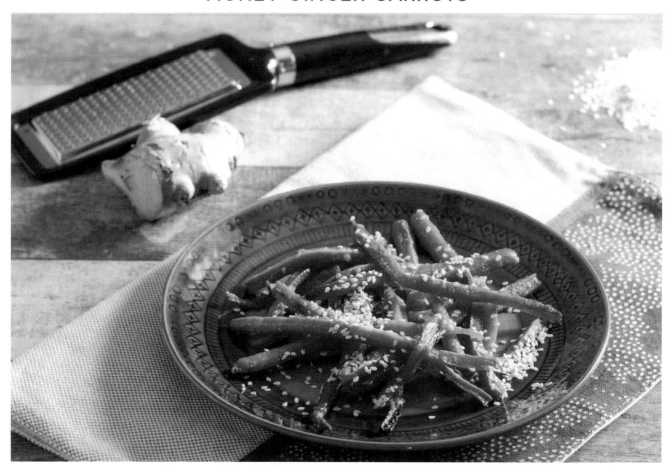

Serves: 1 | **Total Time: 30 minutes**

INGREDIENTS

½ lb carrots, peeled and cut into strips

1 Tbsp fresh ginger, grated

1 Tbsp clover honey*

1 Tbsp olive oil

1 tsp sesame seeds*

sea salt to taste

DIRECTIONS

1. Preheat oven to 400°F.

2. In a large bowl whisk together the olive oil, honey, and fresh ginger. Add the carrots and toss to coat.

3. Spoon the carrots onto a baking sheet.

4. Bake in the oven for 20–25 minutes, until fork tender.

5. Transfer the carrots to a plate. Sprinkle with sesame seeds and serve.

* denotes limited amount—please see yes/no list on page 62

SAUTÉED BOK CHOY

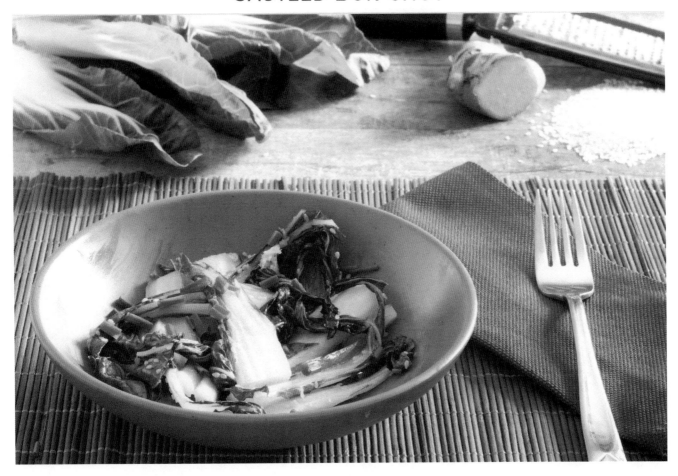

Serves: 2 | **Total Time: 10 minutes**

INGREDIENTS

2 cups (170g) bok choy, washed*

2 scallions, green part only, chopped

1 Tbsp olive oil

1 Tbsp fresh ginger, grated

1 tsp sesame seeds*

sea salt to taste

DIRECTIONS

1 Heat 1 Tbsp of olive oil in a skillet over medium heat.

2 Cut the bok choy in half lengthwise.

3 Add the bok choy and grated ginger to the skillet. Sauté until the bok choy softens and the leaves turn dark green, about 4–6 minutes.

4 Remove from the pan and place in a serving bowl. Garnish with the chopped scallions and sesame seeds. Season with salt to taste and serve.

* denotes limited amount—please see yes/no list on page 62

ROASTED ROOT VEGETABLES

Roasting root vegetables deepens their flavor and is a perfect way to cook them during the autumn and winter months. Simply toss the cut veggies with a bit of oil and sprinkle on your favorite seasonings. Make sure to cut the veggies into chunks of a similar size so they are all done at the same time. The smaller the chunks the faster they'll cook so, if you are in hurry, cut the veggies smaller.

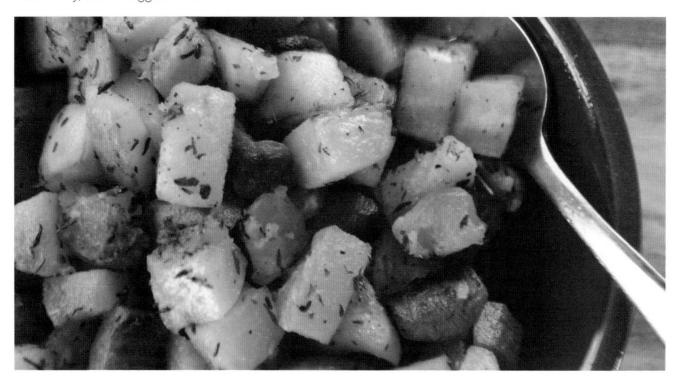

Serves: 6　|　**Total Time: 50—55 minutes**

INGREDIENTS

1 cup rutabaga, cut into ½" cubes

1 cup parsnips, cut into ½" cubes*

1 cup carrots, cut into ½" cubes

¾ cup butternut squash,
　cut into ½" cubes*

2 Tbsp olive oil

1 tsp thyme

DIRECTIONS

1 　Preheat the oven to 350°F

2 　Place cut vegetables in a flat bottomed casserole dish.

3 　Drizzle the olive oil over the veggies and toss them around until they are evenly coated.

4 　Distribute the thyme, herbs de provence, salt & pepper evenly over the vegetables.

5 　Place casserole dish on the middle rack of the preheated oven

6 　Roast the vegetables for 35–40 minutes, stirring once or twice until they are cooked through and beginning to brown slightly.

* denotes limited amount—please see yes/no list on page 62

INDIAN STYLE CABBAGE

For a veggie side dish that comes together quickly, consider this recipe for a spicy cabbage stir-fry with the aroma and flavors of India. I use chili flakes and fresh ginger to add a bit of heat to this dish. Serve with a dollop of Homemade Yogurt (see recipe on page 83) on the side if you want to temper the heat a bit.

Serves: 4 | **Total Time: 18–20 minutes**

INGREDIENTS

4 cups cabbage, shredded*

1 Tbsp Garlic Infused Olive Oil
 (see recipe on page 82)

2 tsp fresh ginger, finely minced

1 tsp turmeric

½ tsp mustard seed

½ tsp garam masala

½ tsp herbs de provence

¼—½ tsp chili flakes,
 (depending on how hot you
 like it)

¼ tsp sea salt

Grinding of pepper

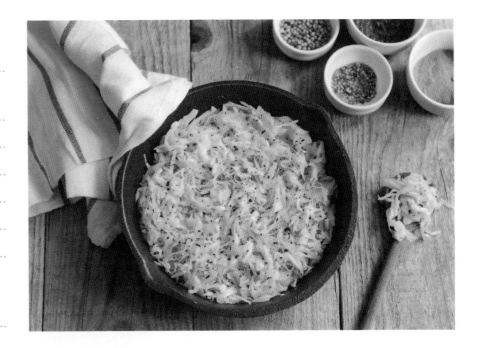

DIRECTIONS

1   Heat oil on medium high in a wok or large frying pan.

2   Add the mustard seed and swirl around in the hot oil for 1 minute then add the garam masala, turmeric, chili flakes and minced ginger and continue to sauté for another 2 minutes.

3   Add the shredded cabbage and cook, stirring continually for at least 5 minutes. This will give you a somewhat crunchy cabbage so simply continue to cook and stir the cabbage a bit longer if you prefer a softer version of cooked cabbage.

* denotes limited amount—please see yes/no list on page 62

Mock Potato Salad

You don't have to give up potato salad! Well, actually you do but you won't mind because you can still enjoy the flavors you love by substituting rutabaga for potato. I know it sounds odd but give it a try. You'll find your mock potato salad tastes so much like the original version that your family and friends won't even know the difference; unless, of course, you tell them!

Serves: 6 | **Total Time: 30 minutes**

INGREDIENTS

4 cups rutabaga, cut into ½" cubes

2 hard boiled eggs

⅓ cup celery, diced small

green parts of 3 scallions, sliced thin

½ cup mayonnaise

1 tsp dijon mustard

sea salt & pepper to taste

sprinkle of paprika

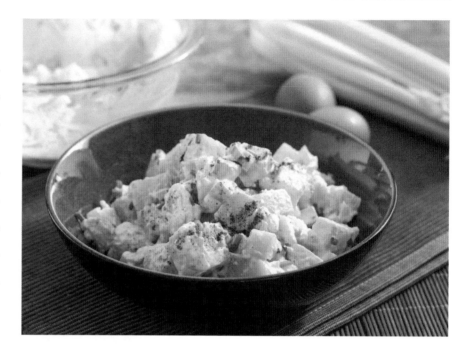

DIRECTIONS

1 Cover rutabaga with water in a large pot and bring to the boil. Adjust heat under the pot and continue to boil until the rutabaga is cooked through but remains firm and is not mushy. Drain and set aside to cool. Chill the cooled rutabaga in the fridge until you are ready to assemble the salad.

2 When it's time to assemble the salad, mash the hard boiled eggs with a fork in a bowl large enough to accommodate all the ingredients.

3 Add the rutabaga, diced celery, sliced scallion and combine with the mayonnaise making sure everything is evenly coated.

4 Add salt and pepper to taste.

5 Serve on a platter or in a bowl garnished with a sprinkle of paprika.

Snacks

I'M HONESTLY NOT MUCH OF A SNACKER. EVER SINCE I SWITCHED FROM THE STANDARD AMERICAN DIET OF PROCESSED FOODS TO A REAL FOOD DIET, I JUST DON'T FEEL THAT HUNGRY BETWEEN MEALS.

Okay, I will admit that it is also because I'm a bit lazy. If I do want a snack, I'll usually just crack open a can of wild caught sardines (awesome source of Omega-3s!) or a can of smoked oysters (great source of Zinc!), sprinkle on some sea salt, and eat it straight out of the can. I know that's probably not everyone's cup of tea so I've included this snack section to give you some ideas of what you can make if you're in a munchy mood or have a party you want to make snacks for.

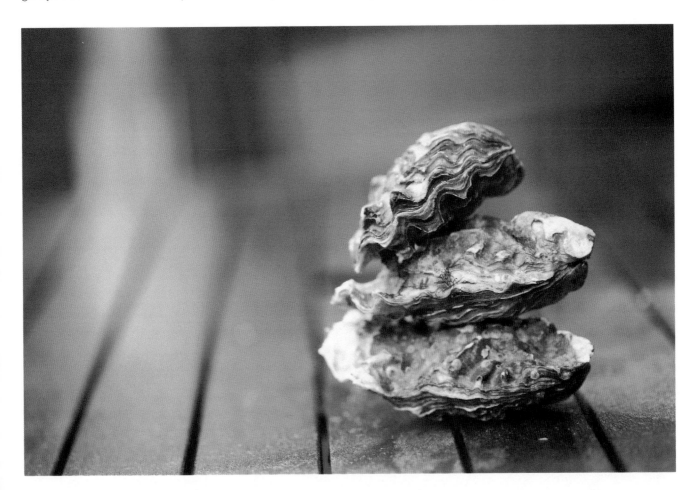

SESAME SEED CRACKERS

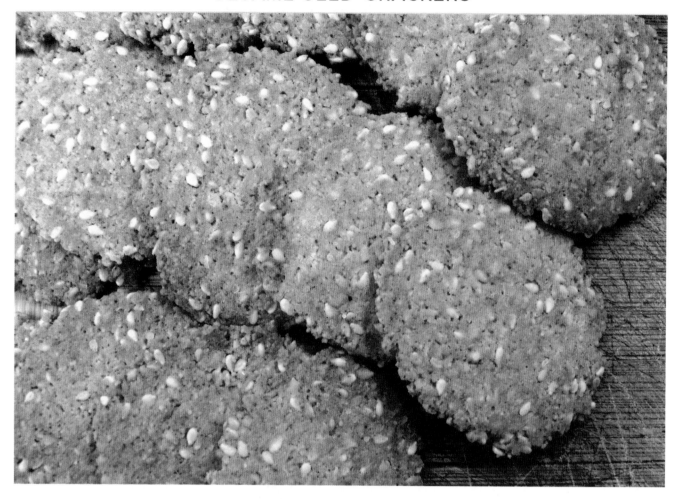

Serves: 8 (makes 32 crackers—4 per portion) | **Total Time: 23–25 minutes**

INGREDIENTS

1 cup almond meal*

4 Tbsp toasted sesame seeds*

1 egg white

1 Tbsp soft butter

¼ tsp sea salt

¼ tsp dijon mustard
  (gluten free, no extra additives)

DIRECTIONS

1   Preheat oven to 325°F

2   Mix together the almond meal and toasted sesame seeds.

3   Mix the egg white, dijon mustard and softened butter into the dry ingredients. Do this by hand making sure the ingredients are all evenly incorporated.

4   Using a teaspoon, make small mounds of the mixture on cookie sheets that have been lined with parchment paper and then flatten gently using the back of a spoon until they're about ¼ inch thick. There should be enough of the cracker mixture to fill two 9″ × 13″ cookie sheets.

* denotes limited amount—please see yes/no list on page 62

LABNEH

Labneh is the Lebanese version of cream cheese that's made using a full fat yogurt. It has a creamy, tangy flavor that you'll love.

Serves: makes 2 cups | **Total Time: 12 hours + 5 minutes prep time**

INGREDIENTS

4 cups full fat Homemade Yogurt
(see recipe on p. 83)

¼ tsp sea salt

DIRECTIONS

1 Line a large sieve with a few layers of cheesecloth so that the cheesecloth hangs over the top edge of the sieve and set the sieve over a deep bowl.

2 Mix together the yogurt and sea salt until the salt is evenly incorporated and place mixture into the lined sieve.

3 Cover with a plate and let the liquid from the yogurt/salt mixture drip into the bowl for a 24 hour period. You will be left with a dense cream cheese that has a mellowed yogurt-like flavor. Refrigerate the Labneh in a tightly covered container until ready to be used.

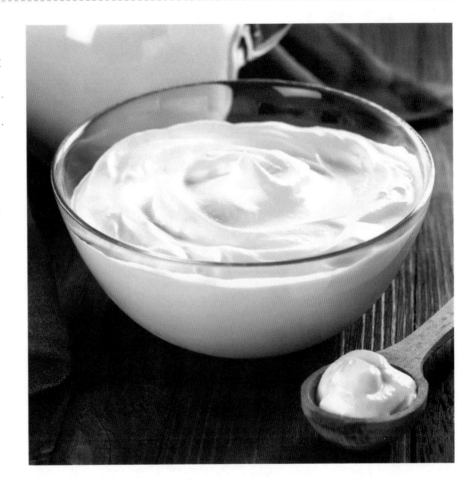

Labneh Herb Dip & Veggie Platter

Customize this dip by using your favourite fresh herbs and serve with raw veggies of choice.

Serves: makes 1 cup | **Total Time: 15 minutes**

INGREDIENTS

1 cup Labneh (see recipe on page 115)

½ Tbsp fresh mint leaves, chopped finely

½ Tbsp fresh thyme, chopped finely

½ Tbsp basil leaves, chopped finely

2 Tbsp Garlic Infused Olive Oil (see recipe on page 82)

1 Tbsp toasted pine nuts*

1 sweet pepper, seeded and cut into strips

2 carrots, cut into small sticks

½ English cucumber, cut into thin wedges

½ cup broccoli, cut into small florets*

DIRECTIONS

1 Combine Labneh, mint, thyme, basil, and 1 tablespoon of the garlic infused olive oil.

2 Place the mixture on a small, flat serving dish. Spread the dip out somewhat, swirling it around to form shallow grooves across the surface.

3 Drizzle the rest of the garlic infused olive oil over the dip.

4 Garnish with toasted pine nuts.

5 Arrange the veggies on a platter and serve next to the dip.

* denotes limited amount—please see yes/no list on page 62

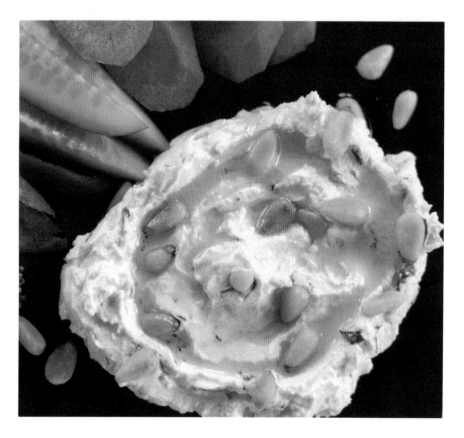

BANANA EGG MUFFINS

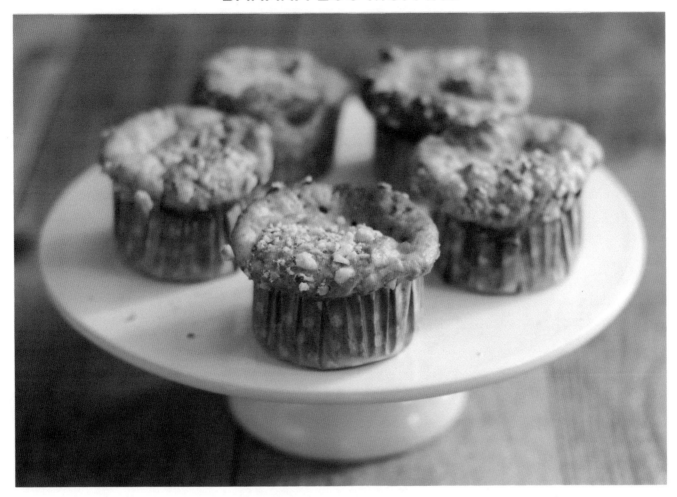

Makes: 8 muffins | **Total Time: 15 minutes**

- -

INGREDIENTS

2 ripe bananas, mashed

4 eggs, beaten

1 Tbsp chopped almonds*

1 tsp vanilla extract

DIRECTIONS

1 Preheat oven to 375°F.

2 In a large bowl mix together the bananas, eggs, almonds and vanilla extract.

3 Pour the batter into 8 muffin cups lined with cupcake liners.

4 Bake in the oven for 12–15 minutes, until the muffins are cooked through.

5 Remove from the oven and serve.

* denotes limited amount—please see yes/no list on page 62

Honey Ginger Hot Wings

Chipotle powder adds heat so feel free to use less for a gentler effect.

Serves: 4 | **Total Time: 35 minutes**

INGREDIENTS

1 lb chicken wings

½ cup honey*

1 ½ Tbsp fresh ginger, peeled & minced

1 Tbsp Garlic Infused Olive Oil (see recipe on page 82)

1 Tbsp lightly toasted sesame seeds

½ tsp chipotle powder

DIRECTIONS

1 Preheat oven to 350°F

2 Wash the chicken wings and pat them dry then place the wings in a bowl large enough to hold them all.

3 Mix the honey, minced ginger, chipotle powder and garlic infused oil together and pour this mixture over the chicken wings, tossing them to make sure they are all evenly coated.

4 Line the wings up on a foil-lined rimmed cookie sheet and sprinkle the toasted sesame seeds over top. Place the pan on the middle rack of the pre-heated oven.

5 Bake for 15 minutes then remove from the oven and, using a brush, baste the wings with some of the honey glaze that has dripped off of the wings and onto the surface of the pan. Be careful not to dislodge the sesame seeds.

6 Return the wings to the oven and bake for another 5–8 minutes until they are a nice golden brown and cooked through.

* denotes limited amount—please see yes/no list on page 62

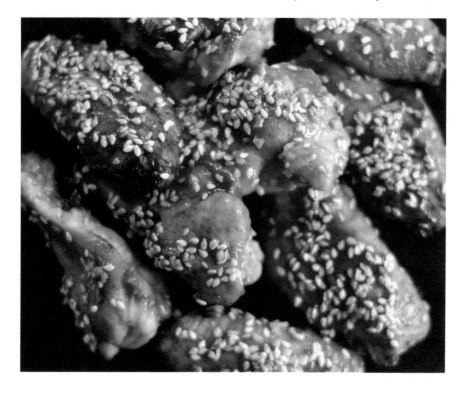

Desserts

SOMETIMES YOU JUST NEED A LITTLE TREAT. IT MAY SEEM LIKE DESSERTS ARE IMPOSSIBLE ON THE SIBO DIET BUT WITH A FEW PIECES OF THE ALLOWABLE FRUIT, A FEW NUTS AND A DASH OF THE ALLOWABLE SWEETENERS YOU CAN MAKE THE OCCASIONAL TREAT THAT YOU'LL ENJOY.

Before my SIBO diagnosis stevia was not a sweetener I would turn to, opting for more natural sweeteners like maple syrup or raw honey. Since maple syrup is not possible with SIBO and only certain types of honey like clover are allowed (which can get a little repetitive), I've included a few recipes which use small amounts of stevia. Of course, you're welcome to skip those recipes or substitute the stevia for what works for you. Green stevia like the one found on our resource page here at www.hollywoodhomestead.com/sibo-solution-resources/ is more natural than it's white powdered counterpart so I would opt for the green one if you can.

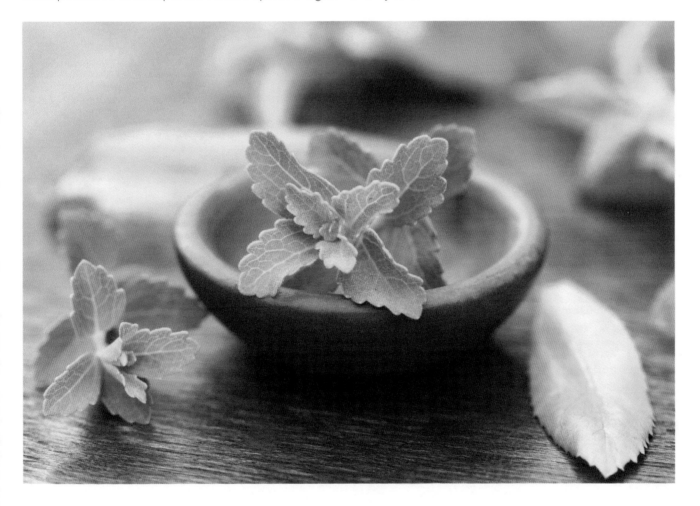

Whipped Banana with Walnut

This is a great alternative to ice cream. It is quick and easy when you just need a little treat!

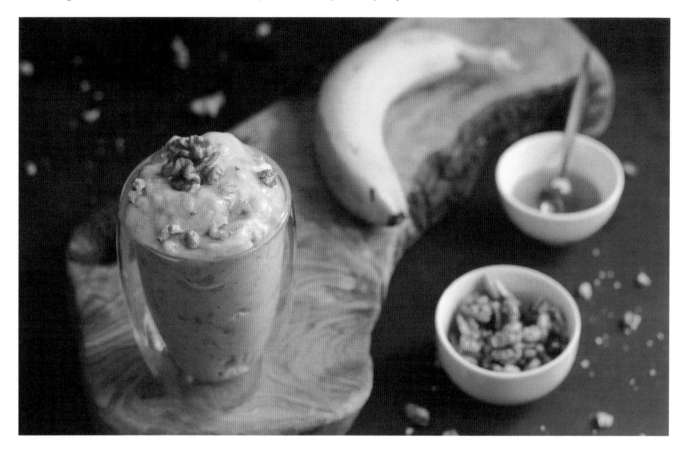

Serves: 1 | **Total Time: 5 minutes**

INGREDIENTS

1 frozen banana

10 walnuts*

Drizzle of clover honey* (about ½ tsp)

Ground cinnamon, to taste

DIRECTIONS

1   Add the walnuts to your food processors bowl. Pulse until nuts are broken into small pieces. Do not over process or it will turn into nut butter.

2   Add the frozen banana and honey.

3   Process for about 30 seconds, until the banana is creamy.

4   Serve immediately and garnish with a banana slice and ground cinnamon, if desired.

* denotes limited amount—please see yes/no list on page 62

HONEY MERINGUE KISS

Light and airy, these little melt-in-the-mouth meringue cookies are sweetened with honey. They go together quickly as there are only two ingredients. However, you need to make these on a day when you will be home for a few consecutive hours as they require a long, slow bake in an oven set at a low temperature. You will notice that these Meringue Kisses made with honey have a more golden hue than traditional meringues, which are usually completely white.

Serves: Makes about 35 little meringue kisses | **Total Time: 2 hours + 5 minutes prep time**

INGREDIENTS

2 egg whites

¼ cup clover honey*

DIRECTIONS

1   Preheat oven to 200°F

2   Place egg whites and honey in a stainless steel bowl. Set the bowl over a saucepan filled with water to a depth of about 3 inches. Place on the bowl and saucepan set-up on a stove-top burner and set it to high. If you have a double boiler, use this!

3   Using a hand-held mixer set to high speed, beat the egg whites while the water beneath the bowl comes slowly to the boiling point.

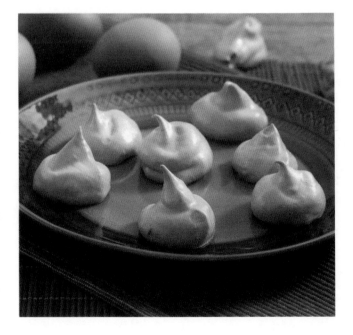

4   Adjust the heat so that the water maintains a slow rolling boil. It's best to wear an oven mitt on the hand holding the bowl as escaping steam could easily scald your fingers.

5   Beat the honey and egg white mixture for five minutes. Turn the burner off. When you remove the bowl from the heat, the mixture will be a slightly off-white golden color and holding stiff peaks.

6   If you have a piping bag, place the beaten egg white mixture into the bag and pipe out 1" diameter kiss-shaped mounds onto a parchment lined cookie sheet. An alternate method is to use a food-safe plastic bag with a small hole cut out of one corner for the piping process. Of course, simply mounding the egg white mixture onto the cookie sheet using a teaspoon is also acceptable (and definitely the easiest method).

7   Place the cookie sheet on the middle rack of a pre-heated oven for 2 hours. When the time is up you will notice that the cookies are still somewhat moist and sticking to the parchment paper. Don't despair, the meringue kisses will dry out and harden as they cool. You will find they are no longer sticking to the parchment paper once they have cooled completely. Store the meringues in an air-tight container at room temperature.

* denotes limited amount—please see yes/no list on page 62

MACAROON COOKIES

When you are in the mood for a little something sweet, a macaroon cookie is hard to beat. I like to bump the flavour up a notch by giving the coconut a light toasting in the oven before mixing up the macaroons. If you decide to go this route, make sure you watch that coconut like a hawk while it's toasting in the oven. It goes from a lovely golden brown to being burnt black in a matter of seconds.

This recipe is for a small batch of cookies as the coconut flour and unsweetened coconut are items that can only be consumed in measured amounts on The SIBO Diet. One cookie equals one serving.

Coconut, although allowed in small quantities on The SIBO Diet can be problematic for some. My recommendation is to try it in small doses and see how it works for you. In other words, try 1 cookie, not a half dozen :)

Serves: 8, 2" cookies; 1 cookie = one serving | **Total Time: 30–33 minutes**

INGREDIENTS

1 cup unsweetened coconut, toasted*

2 egg whites

⅓ cup honey*

⅛ cup coconut flour*

½ tsp vanilla

DIRECTIONS

1 Preheat oven to 350°F

2 Mix the coconut, coconut flour, honey and vanilla together

3 In a separate bowl, whip the egg whites using a hand mixer on high, until they form stiff peaks.

4 Gently fold the egg whites and the coconut mixture together.

5 Line a cookie sheet with parchment paper and divide the batter into mounds with a diameter of about 2".

6 Bake on the middle rack of the oven for 15–18 minutes or until the cookies have turned a golden brown on top. Remove to a wire rack and when cool store the cookies in an airtight container.

* denotes limited amount—please see yes/no list on page 62

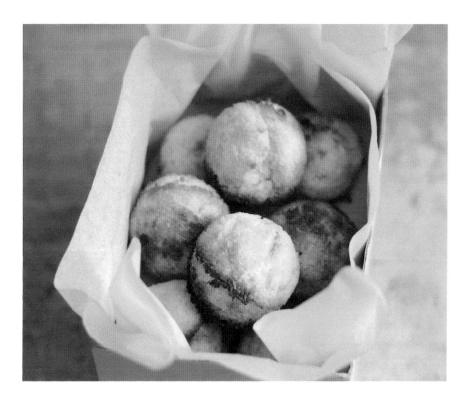

STRAWBERRY PRESERVES

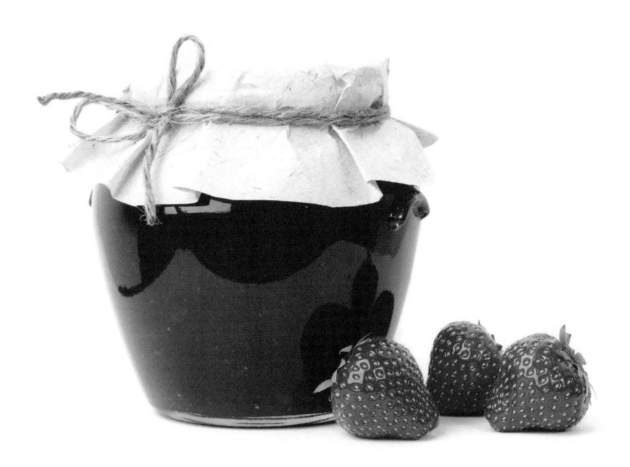

Serves: 2 | **Total Time: 8 minutes**

INGREDIENTS

1 cup frozen strawberries

2 Tbsp honey*

DIRECTIONS

1 In a stainless steel pot over medium-high heat, lightly boil strawberries and honey for 5 minutes.

2 Mash strawberries with a potato masher.

3 Let cool and it's done!

* denotes limited amount—please see yes/no list on page 62

COCONUT ICE CREAM BANANA SPLIT

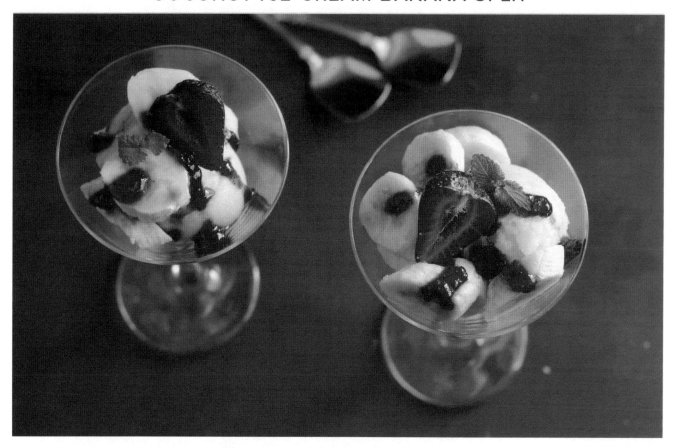

Makes: 8 servings (1 serving = 2 scoops)

Total Time: 15 minutes, cooling time in fridge—4 hours, freezing time will depend on the brand of your ice cream maker!

INGREDIENTS

4 cups coconut milk*

4 egg yolks

½ cup honey*

1 tsp vanilla

Banana slices
    (about ½ banana per split)

Strawberry preserves
    (about 1 Tbsp per split; made
    with honey—see recipe on
    page 123)

DIRECTIONS

1   Gently warm the honey over low heat until it becomes more fluid.

2   Mix coconut milk, egg yolks, and vanilla together in a stainless steel bowl.

3   Slowly add the warm honey into the remaining ingredients while mixing well.

4   Refrigerate the mixture until it is cool (optional but recommended).

5   Place two scoops of ice cream into a bowl, decorate with banana slices and strawberry preserves. There will be enough ice cream for 8 servings. Don't eat more than one serving as the amount of coconut milk you can consume in one sitting on The SIBO Diet is limited.

* denotes limited amount—please see yes/no list on page 62

SHORTBREAD COOKIES

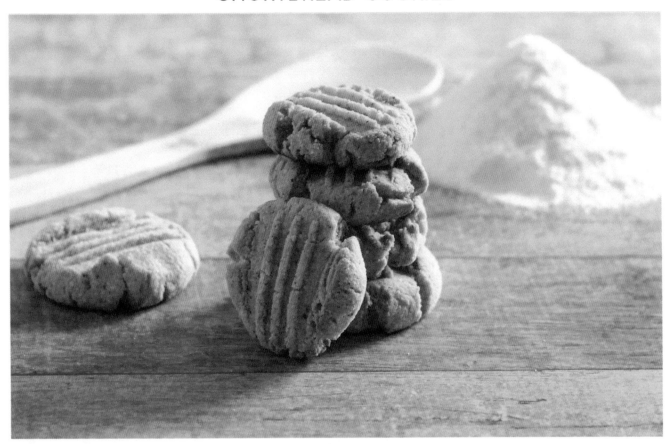

Serves: 3 (2 cookies per serving) | **Total Time: 15 minutes**

INGREDIENTS

6 Tbsp coconut flour*

4 Tbsp butter (or coconut oil), melted

2 Tbsp almond butter*

2 Tbsp honey*

½ tsp vanilla extract

DIRECTIONS

1   Preheat oven to 350°F.

2   Add the ingredients to a large mixing bowl. Use a wooden spoon to mix all the ingredients together until well incorporated.

3   Divide the dough into 6 pieces. Roll each piece into a ball and place on a baking sheet lined with parchment paper.

4   Press each cookie down with a fork, until the top is flattened.

5   Bake in the oven for 7–10 minutes, until the cookies begin to brown.

6   Remove from the oven and allow to cool before serving.

* denotes limited amount—please see yes/no list on page 62

Homemade Yogurt Parfait with Honey and Blueberries

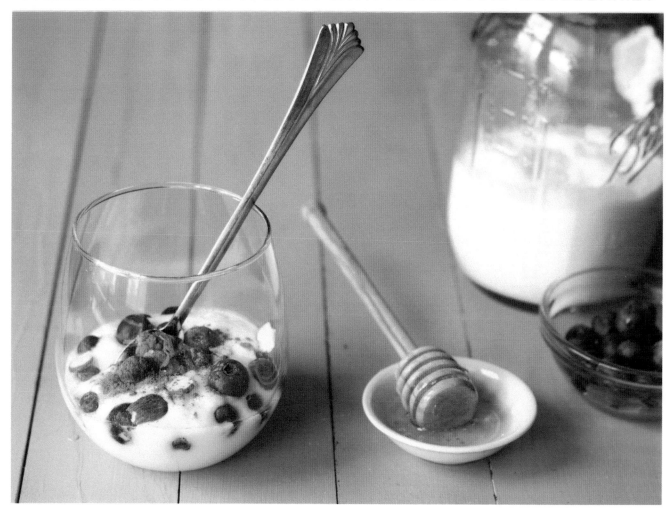

Serves: 2 | **Total Time: 5 minutes**

INGREDIENTS

1 cup plain Homemade Yogurt (24 hour)
  recipe on page 83

40 blueberries*

2 Tbsp clover honey*

2 Tbsp sliced almonds*

DIRECTIONS

1. Add ¼ cup yogurt to a cup.

2. Top with 10 blueberries the blueberries.

3. Top with another ¼ cup yogurt.

4. Top with another 10 blueberries.

5. Add layer of 1 Tbsp. honey and 1 Tbsp. almonds.

6. Repeat for second serving.

* denotes limited amount—please see yes/no list on page 62

COCONUT CUSTARD

Serves: 6 | **Total Time: 40 minutes**

INGREDIENTS

4 eggs

1 can (15oz) full fat coconut milk
(no fillers)*

2–3 Tbsp clover honey, to taste*

1 Tbsp vanilla extract

1 tsp ground cinnamon

¼ tsp ground nutmeg

DIRECTIONS

1. Allow the eggs to rest on the counter at room temperature for 10–15 minutes prior to beginning the cooking process. Preheat the oven to 350 degrees.

2. Prepare 6 ramekins by placing them all on a large baking sheet.

3. Vigorously whisk the eggs in a medium-sized mixing bowl. Set aside.

4. Put coconut milk in saucepan and heat over low heat. Add the honey, vanilla, cinnamon and nutmeg. Stir constantly, until just beginning to simmer.

5. Carefully, and slowly add the milk mixture to the eggs, whisking constantly until well combined and beginning to froth.

6. Pour the mixture evenly into each ramekin, filling them ¾ full.

7. Place in the oven and cook for 30–40 minutes, until the center of the custard if no longer jiggly.

8. Remove and allow to cool for 10–15 minutes. Place in the refrigerator to chill for at least 1 hour.

9. Serve chilled with berries. Enjoy!

* denotes limited amount—please see yes/no list on page 62

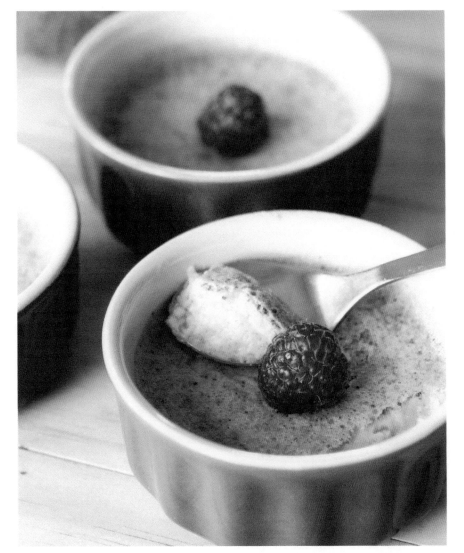

References

1. Kresser, Chris. "SIBO—What Causes It and Why It's so Hard to Treat." *Chris Kresser*. 4 Nov. 2014. Web.

2. Bowen, R. "Gross and Microscopic Anatomy of the Small Intestine." *Vivo Colostate*. 18 Apr. 2000. Web.

3. "Your Digestive System and How It Works." *National Institute of Diabetes and Digestive and Kidney Diseases*. Web.

4. Ruiz, Jr., MD, Atenodoro R. "Small Intestine." *Merck Manual*. 1 Dec. 2014. Web.

5. "Small Intestine."—*MicrobeWiki*. Web. 23 Apr. 2015.

6. O'Hara, Ann, and Fergus Shanahan. "The Gut Flora as a Forgotten Organ." *EMBO Reports*. U.S. National Library of Medicine. Web. 23 Apr. 2015.

7. Reasoner, Jordan. "Everything You Need to Know About SIBO (Small Intestinal Bacterial Overgrowth)." *SCD Lifestyle*. 14 Jan. 2014. Web.

8. Lasich, MD, Christina. "Visceral Hypersensitivity: A Major Source of Abdominal Pain."—*Getting Diagnosed*. 23 July 2012. Web.

9. Siebecker, ND, MSOM, LAc, Allison, and Steven Sandberg-Lewis, ND, DHANP. "Townsend Letter, the Examiner of Alternative Medicine, Online Alternative Medicine Magazine."*Townsend Letter, the Examiner of Alternative Medicine, Online Alternative Medicine Magazine*. 1 Feb. 2013. Web.

10. Jordan, Jo. "Treatment for SIBO and Its Link to Other Diseases | Puristat Digestive Wellness." *Puristat Digestive Wellness*. Web.

11. DiBaise, John K. "Nutritional Consequences of Small Intestinal Bacterial Overgrowth."*Virginia Medicine*. 1 Dec. 2008. Web.

12. "Dietary Supplements: What You Need To Know." *National Institutes of Health*. Web.

13. Mullin, MD, Gerard E. "Gastrointestinal Dysbiosis: What It Is and How to Recognize It."*Functional Medicine*. 1 Feb. 2010. Web.

14. DiBaise, John K. "Nutritional Consequences of Small Intestinal Bacterial Overgrowth."*Virginia Medicine*. 1 Dec. 2008. Web.

15. "Vitamin B$_{12}$." *National Institutes of Health*. 24 June 2011. Web.

16. Foster, Jane A. "Gut Feelings: Bacteria and the Brain." *The Dana Foundation*. 1 July 2013. Web.

17. Kresser, Chris. "Episode 9—the "gut-brain Axis"" *Chris Kresser*. 10 May 2011. Web.

18. Montiel-Castro AJ, González-Cervantes RM, Bravo-Ruiseco G, and Pacheco-López G."The Microbiota-gut-brain Axis: Neurobehavioral Correlates, Health and Sociality." *Frontiers*. 7 Oct. 2013. Web.

19. "Probiotics Send Signals from Your Gut to Your Skin." *Mercola*. 11 Nov. 2010. Web.

20. "Optimizing Your Gut Bacteria Can Help Reduce Acne." *Mercola*. 21 July 2011. Web.

21. Bowe, Whitney, and Alan Logan. "Acne Vulgaris, Probiotics and the Gut-brain-skin Axis—Back to the Future?" *NCBI*. BioMed Central, 31 Jan. 2011. Web.

22. Preidt, Robert. "Many Docs Wrongly Prescribe Powerful Antibiotics: Study—OnHealth."*MedicineNet*. 8 Aug. 2013. Web.

23. Landau, Elizabeth. "Doctors Still Overprescribing Antibiotics." *The Chart*. 3 Oct. 2013. Web.

24. "Food, Farm Animals, and Drugs." *Natural Resources Defense Council*. Web.

25. Amos, Julie-Ann Amos. "Acid Reflux (GERD) Statistics and Facts." *Healthline*. 30 June 2012. Web.

26. "News Flash: Acid Reflux Caused by Too Little Acid, Not Too Much . . . " *Mercola*. 25 Apr. 2009. Web.

27. Kresser, Chris. "The Hidden Causes of Heartburn and GERD." *Chris Kresser*. 1 Apr. 2010. Web.

28. Robillard, Norm. "What Really Causes Acid Reflux and GERD?" *Digestive Health Institute*. 8 July 2014. Web.

29. Dukowicz, Andrew, Brian Lacy, and Gary Levine. "Small Intestinal Bacterial Overgrowth: A Comprehensive Review." *NCBI*. Millennium Medical Publishing, 3 Feb. 2007. Web.

30. McCracken, Sylvie. "How to Treat H. Pylori Naturally." *Hollywood Homestead*. Web.

31. Schmidt, Kyla. "Low Stomach Acid: Cause and Effect." *Kyla Schmidt Is The Digestion Diva*. 1 Apr. 2013. Web.

32. "Hypochlorhydria—Lack of Stomach Acid—Can Cause Lots of Problems."—*DoctorMyhill*. Web.

33. Bowen, R. "The Migrating Motor Complex." *Vivo Colostate*. 22 Oct. 1995. Web.

34. "Dysmotility." *Digestive Disease Center*. Web.

35. Valpone, Amie. "Common Heavy Metals Making You Sick." *The Healthy Apple*. Web.

36. "Heavy Metal Detoxification." *Life Extension*. Web.

37. Noël, Sébastien. «You And Your Gut Flora.» *Paleo Leap*. 28 Dec. 2010. Web.

38. Burkhart, Amy. "What Is Fructose Malabsorption?—Amy Burkhart M.D., R.D." *The Celiac MD*. 22 Feb. 2013. Web.

39. "What Is Crohn's Disease?" *Crohn's & Colitis Foundation of America*. Web.

40. "PubMed for Handhelds/mobiles." *Wikipedia*. Wikimedia Foundation. Web.

41. "The Irritable Bowel Syndrome." *National Center for Biotechnology Information*. U.S. National Library of Medicine. Web.

42. Siebecker, Allison. "SIBO—Small Intestine Bacterial Overgrowth." *SIBO Info*. Web.

43. Hawkey, C.j., Jaime Bosch, Joel E. Richter, Guadalupe Garcia-Tsao, and Francis K. L. Chan. "Textbook of Clinical Gastroenterology and Hepatology." *Google Books*. Wiley-Blackwell. Web.

44. Gastroenterol, Am J. "Normalization of Lactulose Breath Testing Correlates with Symptom Improvement in Irritable Bowel Syndrome. a Double-blind, Randomized, Placebo-controlled Study." *National Center for Biotechnology Information*. U.S. National Library of Medicine, 1 Feb. 2003. Web.

45. Siebecker, Allison. "SIBO—Small Intestine Bacterial Overgrowth." *SIBO Info*. Web.

46. "About Irritable Bowel Syndrome (IBS)." *About IBS*. 2 Apr. 2015. Web.

47. Strudwick, Patrick. "Think You're Bloated by IBS? It Could Just Be Small Intestinal Bacterial Overgrowth and It's Easier to Manage." *Daily Mail*. Associated Newspapers, 21 Jan. 2012. Web.

48. Robillard, Norm. "Crohn's Disease and Diet." *Digestive Health Institute*. 4 Dec. 2013. Web.

49. "Dr. Sidney Valentine Haas Biography." *SC Diet*. Web.

50. Jacob, Aglaée. "Non-responsive Celiac Disease—When Eating Gluten-free Is Not Enough." *Radicata Nutrition*. 15 May 2014. Web.

51. "Why an Endoscopic Biopsy?" *Celiac Disease Foundation*. Web.

52. McCracken, Sylvie. "Is Gluten Free Just a Fad Diet?" *Hollywood Homestead*. Web.

53. McCracken, Sylvie. "Understanding Food Allergies, Sensitivities, and Intolerance." *Hollywood Homestead*. Web.

54. Grace, E., C. Shaw, K. Whelan, and H. J. N. Andreyev. "Small Intestinal Bacterial Overgrowth." *Medscape*. Blackwell Publishing, 1 Jan. 2013. Web.

55. Hicks, Rob. "What Is Small Intestinal Bacterial Overgrowth (SIBO)?" *Web MD*. 4 Mar. 2014. Web.

56. Siebecker, Allison, and Steven Sandberg-Lewis, ND, DHANP. "The Finer Points of Diagnosis, Test Interpretation, and Treatment." *NDNR*. 7 Jan. 2014. Web.

57. "Comprehensive Digestive Stool Test 2 (CDSA2) with Optional Parasitology (CDSA2P)." *Smart Nutrition*. Web.

58. Kresser, Chris. "RHR: Testing for SIBO, Graves Disease, and All about Anemia." *Chris Kresser*. 25 July 2012. Web.

59. "Breath Testing | Johns Hopkins Division of Gastroenterology and Hepatology." *Johns Hopkins Medicine*. Web.

60. Siebecker, Allison. "SIBO Testing." *SIBO Info*. Web.

61. Ghoshal, Uday. "How to Interpret Hydrogen Breath Tests." *NCBI*. Korean Society of Neurogastroenterology and Motility, 11 July 2011. Web.

62. Pimentel, Mark, Robert Gunsalus, Satish Rao, and Husen Zhang. "Methanogens in Human Health and Disease." *Nature*. Nature Publishing Group, 1 Jan. 2012. Web.

63. Fernandes, Judlyn, Angela Wang, Wen Su, Sari Rahat Rozenbloom, Amel Taibi, Elena Comelli, and Thomas Wolever. "Age, Dietary Fiber, Breath Methane, and Fecal Short Chain Fatty Acids Are Interrelated in Archaea-Positive Humans." *The Journal of Nutrition*. 5 June 2013. Web.

64. Basseri, RJ, and K. Chong. "Intestinal Methane Production in Obese Individuals Is Associated with a Higher Body Mass Index." *National Center for Biotechnology Information*. U.S. National Library of Medicine, 8 Jan. 2012. Web.

65. Kresser, Chris. "RHR: SIBO and Methane-What's the Connection?" *Chris Kresser*. 18 Sept. 2014. Web.

66. Siebecker, Allison. "Antibiotics." *SIBO Info*. Web.

67. Marks, Jay. "Small Intestinal Bacterial Overgrowth (SIBO) Causes, Symptoms, Treatment—Small Intestinal Bacterial Overgrowth (SIBO) Treatment—EMedicineHealth." *EMedicineHealth*. 10 Mar. 2014. Web.

68. Turner, Mike. "Antibiotic Resistance: 6 Diseases That May Come Back to Haunt Us." *The Guardian*. 9 May 2014. Web.

69. Quigley, Eamonn, and Rodrigo Quera. "Small Intestinal Bacterial Overgrowth: Roles of Antibiotics, Prebiotics, and Probiotics." *Med Upenn*. 1 Jan. 2006. Web.

70. Neverman, Laurie. "Herbal Antibiotics." *Common Sense Homesteading*. 1 Nov. 2012. Web.

71. Wiviott Tishler, Lori. "Drug-resistant Bacteria a Growing Health Problem." *Harvard Health Blog*. 17 Sept. 2013. Web.

72. Siebecker, Allison. "Herbal Antibiotics." *SIBO Info*. Web.

73. Chedid, V., S. Dhalla, and JO Clark. "Herbal Therapy Is Equivalent to Rifaximin for the Treatment of Small Intestinal Bacterial Overgrowth." *National Center for Biotechnology Information*. U.S. National Library of Medicine, 3 May 2014. Web.

74. McCracken, Sylvie. "Treating SIBO (Part 8): Herbal Antibiotics for SIBO." *Hollywood Homestead*. Web.

75. "The Disappearing Rainforests." *Save the Amazon*. Web.

76. Pimentel, Mark, Yuthana Kong, Meera Bajwa, and Sandy Park. "A 14-Day Elemental Diet Is Highly Effective in Normalizing the Lactulose Breath Test." *Springer Link*. 1 Jan. 2004. Web.

77. Kresser, Chris. "Can a Short-Term Elemental Diet Help Treat SIBO?" *Chris Kresser*. 18 July 2014. Web.

78. Siebecker, Allison. "Elemental Formula." *SIBO Info*. Web.

79. Bowen, R. "The Migrating Motor Complex." *Colorado State*. 22 Oct. 1995. Web.

80. Siebecker, Allison. "Steve Wright Interview." *Chris Kresser*. Web.

81. Dugdale, David. "Peristalsis." *Medline Plus*. U.S. National Library of Medicine, 11 Nov. 2012. Web.

82. Freuman, Tamara. "How Grazing Affects Your Digestive Function." *US News*. U.S.News & World Report, 28 Jan. 2014. Web.

83. Gorard, D.A. "Is the Cyclic Nature of Migrating Motor Complex Dependent on the Sleep Cycle?" *Is the Cyclic Nature of Migrating Motor Complex Dependent on the Sleep Cycle?* 1 May 1998. Web.

84. Siebecker, Allison. "Treatments Strategy for SIBO." *SIBO Info*. Web.

85. Lauritano, EC, M. Gabrielli, and E. Scarpellini. "Small Intestinal Bacterial Overgrowth Recurrence after Antibiotic Therapy." *National Center for Biotechnology Information*. U.S. National Library of Medicine, 1 Aug. 2008. Web.

86. Siebecker, Allison, and Steven Sandberg-Lewis, ND, DHANP. "Small Intestine Bacterial Overgrowth: Often-Ignored Cause of Irritable Bowel Syndrome." *Townsend Letter*. 1 Mar. 2013. Web.

87. Siebecker, Allison. "Dietary Treatments." *SIBO Info*. Web.

88. McCracken, Sylvie. "Treating SIBO (Part 10): Diet for SIBO." *Hollywood Homestead*. Web.

89. Hall, Harriet. "GAPS Diet." *Science-Based Medicine*. 7 May 2013. Web.

90. "Continued Stomach Problems While on GAPS: Healing Journey Part 2." *Mindful Mama*. 25 Aug. 2013. Web.

91. "Diet for IBS and SIBO." *Specialists in Gastroenterology*. Web.

92. Siebecker, Allison. "Prevention." *SIBO Info*. Web.

93. Grace, E., C. Shaw, and K. Whelan. "Small Intestinal Bacterial Overgrowth." *Medscape*. Blackwell Publishing, 1 Jan. 2013. Web.

94. "Small Intestine Bacterial Overgrowth." *The Liberated Kitchen*. 5 Mar. 2013. Web.

95. McCracken, Sylvie. "What Is Leaky Gut Syndrome?" *Hollywood Homestead*. Web.

96. "Hypochlorhydria—Lack of Stomach Acid—Can Cause Lots of Problems."—*DoctorMyhill*. Sarah Myhill Limited, 16 Jan. 2015. Web.

97. Kresser, Chris. "How Too Much Omega-6 and Not Enough Omega-3 Is Making Us Sick." *Chris Kresser*. 8 May 2010. Web.

98. Sisson, Mark. "Why the Omega-3/Omega-6 Ratio May Not Matter After All." *Marks Daily Apple*. 6 Aug. 2014. Web.

99. "The Best Oils." *Mendosa*. 16 Sept. 2008. Web.

100. Gunnars, Kris. "How to Optimize Your Omega-6 to Omega-3 Ratio." *Authority Nutrition*. 7 Nov. 2013. Web.

101. "Checking Your Oil: The Definitive Guide to Cooking with Fat." *Caveman Doctor*. 27 May 2012. Web.

102. McCracken, Sylvie. "How to Make Homemade Ghee." *Hollywood Homestead*. Web.

103. "Why Grassfed Animal Products Are Better." *Mercola*. Web.

104. Leschin-Hoar, Clare. "Why Farmed Salmon Is Losing Its Omega-3 Edge." *Time*. Time, 8 Dec. 2014. Web.

105. Siebecker, Allison. "The Second Opinion Series." *The Digestion Sessions*. 8 Nov. 2014. Web.

106. Horne, Steven, and Thomas Easley. "Natural Therapy for SIBO." *Modern Herbal Medicine*. Web.

107. Shepherd, Sue, and Peter Gibson. "Food, FODMAPs and IBS: What to Eat and What to Avoid." *Australian Healthy Food Guide*. 1 Sept. 2011. Web.

108. McCracken, Sylvie. "How to Make Gelatin-Rich Bone Broth." *Hollywood Homestead*. Web.

109. McCracken, Sylvie. "What Is Histamine Intolerance (and What Can You Do about It)." *Hollywood Homestead*. Web.

Notes

63819657R00074

Made in the USA
Lexington, KY
18 May 2017